Palgrave Studies in Science and Popular Culture

Series Editor
Sherryl Vint
Department of English
University of California
Riverside, CA, USA

This book series seeks to publish ground-breaking research exploring the productive intersection of science and the cultural imagination. Science is at the centre of daily experience in twenty-first century life and this has defined moments of intense technological change, such as the Space Race of the 1950s and our very own era of synthetic biology. Conceived in dialogue with the field of Science and Technology Studies (STS), this series will carve out a larger place for the contribution of humanities to these fields. The practice of science is shaped by the cultural context in which it occurs and cultural differences are now key to understanding the ways that scientific practice is enmeshed in global issues of equity and social justice. We seek proposals dealing with any aspect of science in popular culture in any genre. We understand popular culture as both a textual and material practice, and thus welcome manuscripts dealing with representations of science in popular culture and those addressing the role of the cultural imagination in material encounters with science. How science is imagined and what meanings are attached to these imaginaries will be the major focus of this series. We encourage proposals from a wide range of historical and cultural perspectives.

More information about this series at
http://www.palgrave.com/gp/series/15760

Lulu Le Vay

Surrogacy and the Reproduction of Normative Family on TV

palgrave
macmillan

Lulu Le Vay
London, UK

Palgrave Studies in Science and Popular Culture
ISBN 978-3-030-17569-6 ISBN 978-3-030-17570-2 (eBook)
https://doi.org/10.1007/978-3-030-17570-2

Cover image: Rob Lewine/Getty Images
Cover design by eStudio Calamar

This Palgrave Macmillan imprint is published by the registered company Springer Nature Switzerland AG
The registered company address is: Gewerbestrasse 11, 6330 Cham, Switzerland

For my mother Sonja Le Vay and my dear friend Zoe Smith.
I will never forget you.

Preface and Acknowledgements

Why Surrogacy?

I often get asked what sparked my interest in surrogacy, deemed an unusual subject for a book about its representation on TV. In 2010, after a decade of ongoing reproductive health issues which resulted in numerous surgeries (and finally a full hysterectomy in 2016) my gynaecologist informed me that if I wanted children 'of my own'—i.e. of a genetic connection—I should consider surrogacy. I was stunned, as this was something that I had never considered, or known that much about. As a consumer of TV and popular culture, the only reference I had at this point was that *Sex and the City* star Sarah Jessica Parker had engaged a surrogate to produce twin girls in 2009. This was a story that had been splashed across the popular press, which I had read. Since this time, of course, a plethora of celebrities have engaged a surrogate to help them have children, a reproductive choice which continues to stimulate column inches. Singer Elton John and David Furnish, and actor Nicole Kidman and Keith Urban, to name just a few, have expanded their families through this practice. American TV personalities Giuliana and Bill Rancic's surrogacy tale steered the narrative of their hit reality TV show *Giuliana & Bill*, which is explored in this project. At the time of writing Kim Kardashian and Kanye West have just announced they are expecting their fourth child—the second child to be carried by a surrogate. As Kim gushed on her social media platforms after the birth of their first surrogate baby Chicago in January 2018: 'Having a gestational carrier was so special for us… she made our dreams of expanding a family come true' (Msn 2019). What I found intriguing is that the core driving force of the fast-growing surrogacy practice appears to be the preservation of the genetic tie. Any other formations of family outside of this, such as fostering or adoption (unless you're Madonna) are seen as having less value. I wanted to try and make sense of this reproductive desire and what impact this might have on the future of family, why the media appear to be so fascinated by it, and to try and get some understanding of the industry that profits from it.

I'm not a wealthy celebrity with a disposable income. However, I have friends who have managed to fund IVF and egg donation to help them build their families. I have also encountered people in my circles who know someone who has turned to surrogacy. What this indicates is that the industry does reach regular folk outside of celebrity circles. Despite this, surrogacy was never something I wished to pursue. I just didn't want children *that* much. Even so, my journalistic curiosity inspired me to explore how the practice worked, primarily in Britain. As it turned out, communications with a surrogacy agency revealed that I would not be able to get the parental order for the child—the document that would enable me to become the legally named parent—as I was unattached. As the email from the agency representative explained: 'I'm afraid that, as a single person, surrogacy in the UK is not an option for you'. This infuriated me so much I wrote a feature about it for *The Independent* (Le Vay 2010), which involved interviews with a specialist surrogacy law firm and the medical director of the London Women's Clinic. Both parties agreed that the surrogacy laws in Britain were out of date and needed revising. After this article was published, all noticed surrogacy storylines everywhere, not just fodder for gossip showbiz headlines, but on mainstream TV shows.

Why TV?

The media has been, and still is, an integral part of my life. Telling stories—and listening to them—through various forms became my career. I've worked as a journalist for twenty years across print and broadcasting. Now, in my forties, I've embraced my bookish leanings and have 'come out' as an academic—I am now a proud sociologist and media scholar. Better late than never.

As a human being living on the planet right now—at a specific time and in a certain place—I am a fascinated by modern life and the culture that eddies around it, which is why I got into journalism in the first place. I've been a consumer of TV since I was a kid, and in my late twenties I spent a short time working as a TV researcher on a late-night music show. Although the *production* of TV content is a crucial topic to explore, I wanted to focus on its *reception* with audiences, as my interest lies with finding out what people think about the world around them—and TV is a powerful cultural artefact that must be scrutinised.

I grew up in the 1970s when as a family we would huddle around the one crappy TV set in the kitchen with a temperamental aerial to watch *Doctor Who* (1963–1989) or *Tales of the Unexpected* (1979–1988), which I would be so terrified of that I would end up hiding behind the sofa, peeking through trembling fingers. Despite this, I still loved watching these shows. The music still makes my neck hair tingle. I also remember my older brothers, without my mother's knowledge, letting me stay up late to watch cult American stoner movie *Up in Smoke* (1978), a comedy which features two men smoking giant spliffs. Through watching TV, I learnt about life outside the sleepy East Sussex countryside. In 2019, watching programmes and films on digital on-demand services like Netflix, in the middle of the Cotswolds or the Australian outback, wouldn't be much different.

My job in this book is to unpack what a number of TV shows featuring surrogacy storylines are saying about reproduction, family structures and motherhood, with the help of a number of focus group participants. I believe stories matter. I believe audience work matters. I believe, following others in the field, that opening up a dialogue between the text and audience is a vital method by which to produce valuable data.

As part of this explorative journey I am also curious to determine what it was about the genre of the show that made me hide behind the sofa as a kid, yet still give me pleasure in the viewing process? Emotion and affect in relation to TV are important factors to consider, which I explore through an examination of how emotion is structured in the shows and interpreted by viewers. This will include a rigorous analysis of the character constructions, dialogue, style of filming, camera angles and the art of the close-up. Have you ever wondered what techniques make you reach for the tissues or throw a blanket over your head? Ever questioned what it was about a specific character that made you feel an empathetic connection? Clever stuff, this TV lark.

It is common that research projects are inspired by personal experiences—and/or sympathies with a specific area—which should be acknowledged as the project's starting point (Taylor in Wetherell et al. 2001). Therefore, I acknowledge the conversation with my gynaecologist in his consulting room and the times hiding behind the sofa as pivotal moments in my research career, and this book's starting point.

Acknowledgements

I want to express my deepest gratitude to those people who helped make this book happen. Foremost, I want to thank the participants who took part in this project. Without them, this book would not have been possible. I also want to thank my colleagues Beverley Skeggs, Rebecca Coleman, Jo Littler and Kirstyn Gorton for all their constructive feedback on this work as it developed and inspiring me to keep going with it. I will also be eternally grateful to Hannah Le Vay and Jessica Carlisle for their close reading of the manuscript, and to all my wonderful mates for all their consistent encouragement. Despite the obstacles, we made it to the finish line.

London, UK Lulu Le Vay

References

Le Vay, Lulu. 2010. "Why Can't I Have a Baby on My Own?" *The Independent*, May 20.

Msn. 2019. "Kim Kardashian West Thanks Surrogate After Baby's Birth." Available from: https://www.msn.com/enca/entertainment/celebrity/kim-kardashian-west-thanks-surrogate-after-babys-birth/ar-AAuSqky?li=AAjnRI7. Accessed 20 February 2019.

Wetherell, Margaret, Stephanie Taylor, and Simeon Yates. 2001. *Discourse as Data*. Los Angeles: Sage.

About This Book

This book explores representations and responses to surrogacy on TV and film. It examines how conventional notions of 'the proper family' are reproduced. Through textual analysis and audience work, this research explores how conventional ideals of family are constructed, and how female viewers interpret such values. A specific focus is on how narratives are articulated through genre devices, and how particular televisual techniques shape audience perception.

Through textual and empirical methods, this book demonstrates how dominant textual narratives are steered by constructing heterosexual infertile characters as non-normative, in need of transformation into genetic mothers through surrogacy, or natural pregnancy enabled by heterosexual love. Same-sex parenting and homosexuality are articulated as more acceptable when positioned within compulsory monogamy. Through the lens of queer theory, conventional notions of family, motherhood and femininity are exposed, as any positions outside of this ideal are portrayed as failing to comply.

The research was conducted through three focus groups of women, consisting of mothers and non-mothers. Clips from popular mainstream texts featuring surrogacy storylines across sitcom, soap, reality TV and film were shown. Despite the hetero-norms that drive the narratives in the texts, the audience data revealed desires to see alternative happy endings that show infertile female characters more positively, and which recognise alternative formations of kinship situated outside of heteronormative monogamy and the genetic tie. The research respondents consider alternatives *as* meaningful, if not *more* reflective of contemporary structures of family.

This research reveals the temporal gap between mainstream texts, which uphold the white, heteronormative, genetically reproduced family as the ideal, at a time when forms of families are continually diversifying, and when more women are choosing alternative life paths outside of marriage and motherhood.

Praise for *Surrogacy and the Reproduction of Normative Family on TV*

"Drawing on a rich archive of feminist scholarship, this timely and original analysis of repro-TV dramas and new ways of baby-making unpacks the normative scripting of (in)fertility journeys and makes a powerful and persuasive case for new plotlines in popular culture and beyond."

—Sarah Franklin, *University of Cambridge, UK*

"When and how did the foetus become a commodity? When and how did motherhood become sexualised? When did having children become a socially necessary compulsion? This book offers a great read to answer these and many more questions, showing how a sensationalised emotional space of anxiety, insecurity, desperation and incompleteness is produced by TV to shape our expectations of future family life. But does it succeed?"

—Beverley Skeggs, *London School of Economics, UK*

"This book is a significant and indeed seminal volume on the representation of surrogacy and third party reproduction on screen. The ways in which the author and the audience make sense of the depiction of surrogates, intended parents and the much longed for biological child is a must read for those researching from within the fields of motherhood, film, television and media studies."

—Rebecca Feasey, *Bath Spa University, UK*

"Sparkily written, perceptive and illuminating, this is a fascinating and original contribution to the burgeoning academic literature on representations of family and motherhood. Lulu le Vay's book incisively analyses both the place of surrogacy in contemporary culture and TV's fascination with it. In the process, it argues convincingly that both media and academia cultures need to make much more space for the diversity of what 'a family' can mean."

—Jo Littler, *City, University of London, UK*

"Le Vay's timely book explores representations of surrogacy and motherhood in the media. Through a series of close analyses of TV programmes such as *The New Normal and Modern Family* and films such *Baby Mama* and *Rules of Engagement*, she explores not only the anxieties surrounding infertility and the impact of reproductive technologies, but also the ways that these anxieties reflect the changing shape of family in modern life. Drawing on queer, affect and feminist theory, and through the use of focus groups, Le Vay offers an original and compelling interpretation of issues around surrogacy in popular culture."

—Kristyn Gorton, *York University, UK*

Contents

About the Author

Lulu Le Vay is a former journalist who has had work published in *The Independent*, *The New Statesman* and *The Guardian* as well as in music and lifestyle titles such as The Face, Sleazenation, Jockey Slut, Dazed and i-D. She has interviewed Missy Elliot in Puerto Rico, Barry White in San Diego, and has discovered new sides of Brooklyn and Ibiza on two wheels for Cycling Active magazine.

As well as being a writer, Lulu is also an educator and DJ. Alongside lecturing in music and media at a number of London universities, Lulu's passion for music and love of travelling has led her to DJ in Ibiza, Los Angeles, Chicago and Miami. She can also be seen performing at some of London's hippest happenings and venues, from the Tate Modern on Bankside to The Groucho in Soho.

A change of path from journalism into academia led Lulu to attain a Ph.D. in Sociology from Goldsmiths, University of London, in 2018.

List of Figures

CHAPTER 1

Introduction: Family in Crisis—The Rise of Surrogacy and Its Impact on Popular Culture

What Is Surrogacy?

Before we get into the juicy bits about what this book is about, a good place to start is to explain what surrogacy actually is. Traditional surrogacy is when a surrogate uses her own egg, which is fertilised though either IVF or artificial insemination. Gestational surrogacy is when the surrogate carries a foetus that she is not genetically related to which is implanted into the uterus via embryo transfer. Most commonly the foetus is genetically connected to one or both intended parents. Transnational surrogacy is a form of medical tourism when hopeful parents turn to the Global South to engage a foreign surrogate labourer. A glossary of terms can be found in Appendix A. The fees involved vary dependent on what the legal framework is for each country. For instance, in Britain the only permitted arrangement is altruistic surrogacy, where surrogates are only allowed to claim for medical expenses, and no further monetary compensation. Whereas in California, where commercial surrogacy is legal and agencies brokering these services are aplenty, women carrying the genetic offspring for others are rewarded for their services, the process costing in the region of £100,000. Variations in the law and processes will be explained further on and addressed throughout the book.

L. Le Vay, *Surrogacy and the Reproduction of Normative Family on TV*, Palgrave Studies in Science and Popular Culture,
https://doi.org/10.1007/978-3-030-17570-2_1

Reproductive Technologies and the Discourse of Desperation

According to recent population surveys, more women in Britain (Ons.gov.org) and America (Census.gov) are childless in modern times, and fertility is dwindling. The Human Fertilisation and Embryo Authority (HFEA) report that between 1991 and 2016 there have been over one million IVF cycles in British licensed clinics, resulting in 20,028 births. Since 2014, frozen IVF treatment cycles have increased by 39%. Since 1978, four decades after the birth of IVF miracle Louise Brown, the European Society of Human Reproduction (ESHRE) claim that over eight million babies have been born through IVF worldwide. Surrogacy is also on the rise, which involves embryo transfer through IVF. A report by Children and Family Court Advisory and Support Service (CAFCASS) has revealed that since 2013 surrogacy rates have increased in Britain by 90%, the numbers of Parental Order applications received by the courts having reached in the region of 300 in 2018. However, as CAFCASS highlight, these numbers are not precise, as they are subject to possible errors with data entry and processing. A Parental Order is the legal documentation that transfer rights of the child from the surrogate to the IP (intended parents). It is common that one IP has a genetic connection to the child, which differentiates the process from adoption, which the Ministry of Justice claims is continuing a downward turn.

As stated by the Centers for Disease Control and Prevention (CDC), in 1999, 727 gestational carrier cycles were recorded in America which rose to 3432 in 2013. Elsewhere, a UN-backed study in 2012 has revealed that in India, where transnational surrogacy has been hugely popular, there were an estimated 3000 clinics, generating an income of $400 million per year (Choudhary 2015). In 2015 the Indian government banned all international surrogacy arrangements, the bulk of this vast income. The service, which was once open to unmarried couples and single people, gay or straight, is now only available to Indian heterosexual married couples.

Reproduction through the growing commercial surrogacy industry, during a time in history when infertility is on the rise, has become a site for anxiety, a complex issue that has inspired debate from all corners of society. As Miranda Davies (2017) highlights in her work on transnational surrogacy: 'it is not surprising that for journalists, scholars, rights activists, would-be-parents and indeed anyone interested in the evolution of humankind in the twenty-first century, the popularity of transnational surrogacy has become something of a "hot topic"' (2017, 1). Such a hot topic has been explored in cultural representations as well as reflected in inconsistent legal frameworks globally. For example, during the period of this research project commercial surrogacy for foreigners has been banned in not only India, but Thailand, Nepal and Cambodia. Altruistic surrogacy is legal in Britain, Australia, Greece, Mexico and Malaysia. This is where the surrogate is compensated not through a fee, but through reasonable expenses. Families Through Surrogacy (Everingham 2017) declares that due to recent legal changes, commercial surrogacy has shifted to Greece, Laos and the Ukraine. This report also outlines that overwhelmingly, whether commercial or altruistic surrogacy, the practice is only available to heterosexual couples—America, Canada, Kenya, Laos and Mexico being the only countries where 'all' types of commissioning intended parents are welcome.

The laws surrounding surrogacy are complex, unstable, and continually changing, and ethical debates and news stories continue to make the headlines, primarily with theories of exploitation, tales of hope, heartbreak, lost and won court battles, and denied citizenship cases. One of the most impactful surrogacy reports to break during the development of this project was the Thai surrogacy case in 2014, which dominated global headlines. It was claimed that an Australian couple refused to take home their downs syndrome genetic son Gammy, preferring to keep his heathy twin sister, Pipah. The Thai surrogate mother was given legal custody of Gammy. The drama of the case created a powerful narrative which attracted the global spotlight.

As Sarah Franklin (1990) has argued: 'popular representations are a powerful force in the social world and cultural construction of reproduction' (1990, 227). The Gammy news story follows a similar narrative to her analysis of how infertility and IVF treatment was represented in the popular press two decades ago—which indicates not much has changed. In this work she proposes that discourses of desperateness—which she claims are derived from popular romance narratives—are central to these stories, through the structuring of binaries. As she explains: 'It's a story of winners or losers, of happy endings for some and hopelessness for others... Most importantly, however, it's a story of "desperateness"' (1990, 204). This work provides a core foundation for this book, which I have drawn upon to explore contemporary TV shows with surrogacy storylines, a main component of which includes narratives of infertility.

The Gammy surrogacy story connected with the public through the heart-breaking tale of a woman's infertility and a couple's desperation for a child. The winner/loser binary emerged through the divisions of the twins—one healthy, one disabled; one wanted, one rejected. The ending of the story was framed by a twist on the conventional romance narrative—the surrogate fell in love with the baby she was carrying, which the genetic parents didn't want, and kept him. The genetic parents were portrayed as unfit, and surrogacy as a commercial practice was depicted as unethical, immoral and hazardous to children. It came as no surprise that Thailand changed its surrogacy laws in the aftermath of the media outrage.

Surrogacy on TV—The Selection Process

Surrogacy has captured the popular imagination through its growing visibility in popular culture, particularly over the last decade. Not just through the media spectacle of new stories and celebrities' personal lives, but through a growing number of popular fictional and reality TV shows.

This book contributes to the field of television scholarship by exploring representations of surrogacy on TV and film, through textual analysis and audience work. To do this, TV shows featuring surrogacy storylines had to be identified and analysed, and then clips from a selection of these shows shown to and discussed by three focus groups of women. The first phase of this research required compiling a list of these shows, across a wide breadth of genres. I then had the tricky job of getting access to as many of these shows as I could. I limited the timescale of the TV search to 1988 onwards, due to the focus being on gestational surrogacy—that is, when the surrogate is not genetically linked the foetus—enabled through advancements in reproductive technologies at this time. I argue throughout the book that these developments have influenced television and film narratives. In accord with media scholar Kelly Oliver (2012), whose work on the images of pregnancy in Hollywood film is a recommended accompaniment to this book, films (and in this project's case, TV shows) should be examined within the cultural and technological contexts of their time. With this in mind, it was also decided to focus on texts from 2004 onwards, within a contemporary time frame. This was not only to keep within the most recent developments of reproductive technologies over the last decade, but also to hope that participants might have some familiarity with the texts and the practice of surrogacy, which would support the discussion. For instance, in ten years' time if a similar project emerges, it is likely to present some different examples, with different findings. Who knows what reproductive technological developments will surface in the future?

The restrictions I encountered on my investigative journey were primarily due to money and access. It transpired that some DVDs of the documentaries I wanted to obtain were expensive—many of which lacked English subtitles—and talk shows such as *Oprah!* were just not available. Although the lack of access was frustrating, the result was that the research design became more focused. Therefore, I created a core library of genre categories—soap opera, film, documentary, sitcom, drama and reality TV. A discussion of genre as an ever-evolving field is discussed further on. The initial content of this library contained a number of shows. In sitcom: *Rules of Engagement* (E!, 2007–2013), *The New Normal* (NBC, 2012–2013) and *Friends* (NBC, 1994–2004). In soap opera: *Coronation Street* (ITV, 1960–present) and *Doctors* (BBC, 2000–present). In TV drama: *Brothers & Sisters* (ABC, 2006–2011), *The Good Wife* (CBS, 2009–2016), *Drop Dead Diva* (Lifetime, 2009–2014) and *Grey's Anatomy* (ABC, 2005–present). In reality TV: *Giuliana & Bill* (E!, 2009–2014), *The Little Couple* (TLC, 2009–2016), *Kourtney & Kim Take Miami* (E!, 2009–2013) and *The Only Way Is Essex* (ITV2, 2010–2014; ITVBe, 2014–present). In documentary: *Google Baby* (HBO, 2009), *Paternal Instinct* (Cinemax, 2005), *Breeders: A Subclass of Women?* (CBC, 2014), *Was That My Baby Crying?* (NDTV, 2008), *Addicted to Surrogacy* (Channel 4, 2009), *Naître Père* (De Films En Aiguille, 2013) and *Made in India* (PBS, 2010). In film: *The Brothers Solomon* (Revolution Studios, 2007), *Baby Mama* (Relativity Media, 2008), *The Surrogacy Trap* (Incendo, 2013), *The Surrogate* (ABC, 1995), *Filhaal* (Dharma, 2002) and *Born to Be Sold* (Ron Samuels, 1981). In miniseries: *Baby M* (ABC, 1998).

Over the summer of 2014, I watched a *lot* of telly, as a close viewing process was required. This procedure and in-depth notetaking allowed me to identify patterns of dominant ideologies that emerged in the narratives, such as the ideologies of completeness (the value of motherhood and femininity through fertility), natural reproduction (normative family), romance (which enables normative family), heterosexuality (happiness attached to the heterosexual couple dyad and the nuclear family) and whiteness (value of the white genetic child, fear of miscegenation, reproducing the white nuclear family). In addition to this, a close examination of the genre techniques was also recorded, as an important part of this research was to explore how, if at all, such techniques shape the audience's perception of the practice—which I was able to determine through the viewing sessions.

After this close analysis I decided to exclude documentary and drama. This was to narrow the focus for the book even further; to allow a much deeper examination of the more mainstream shows with stronger surrogacy storylines. Therefore, the final shows that made the cut for the book include American sitcoms *Rules of Engagement* (E!, 2007–2013) and *The New Normal* (NBC, 2012–2013), American reality TV show *Giuliana & Bill* (E!, 2009–2014), British soap opera *Coronation Street* (ITV, 1960–present) and Hollywood film *Baby Mama* (2008). A full description of these shows is set out in Appendix B. Interestingly, after this book's research was completed, a number of popular TV programmes and films with surrogacy-related storylines materialised, particularly within the TV drama category. These include multiple award-winner *The Handmaid's Tale* (Hulu, 2017–present)and *Top of the Lake: China Girl* (Sundance BBC, 2017), both of which star Elisabeth Moss of *Mad Men* (AMC, 2007–2015) fame.

Contemporary TV Drama Within the Context of Reproductive Politics

The Handmaid's Tale is a contemporary reworking of Margaret Atwood's (1985) dystopian novel, which tells the story of a fundamentalist regime in America who apprehend fertile women due to plummeting birth rates and make them the property of the state to reproduce. Due to this show's popularity the Hulu network have considered the potential for it to be extended to ten seasons, moving beyond its original plot.[1] Although originally situated in a future that is dehumanising for women, one which was once considered unthinkable, the programme reflects the current state of contemporary American politics. At the time of the show's production Donald Trump's administration has threatened women's reproductive rights by withdrawing funds from healthcare organisation Planned Parenthood, resulting in women having less access to birth control and abortions—not just in America, but globally. Furthermore, with Trump's appointment of anti-abortion judges to the Supreme Court, women's reproductive rights have been put further under threat, the overturning of the landmark *Roe Vs Wade* decision in 1973, which allowed women to have safe and legal abortions across America, becoming increasingly likely. It is unsurprising, then, that *The Handmaid's Tale* has resonated so deeply with viewers. In the same year Sydney-based *Top of the Lake: China Girl* (2017) materialised, the first popular drama to address transnational surrogacy in Australia, where gestational surrogacy is illegal. The narrative follows Australian couples illegally contracting Thai prostitutes, who eventually flee back home with the intended parents' precious cargo on board. This is the first fictional articulation of transnational surrogacy to have appeared on our screens. The storyline tackles not just the ethical and moral dilemmas of the practice but spotlights the precarious outcomes of volatile legal frameworks that can leave intended parents broke (and heartbroken), and genetic offspring left in citizenship limbo. As fertility specialist Bronwyn Devine of leading Australian clinic Monash IVF states: 'The [Australian] system is broken… Compensated surrogacy in a regulated environment is now essential to protect Australian couples and surrogates as well as reduce exploitation of women overseas' (Devine 2017).

Although drama was omitted from the original research phase, it is important to acknowledge these shows. Therefore, they are discussed throughout the book, but not with as much depth as I would have liked, as frustratingly they did not exist when the bulk of the research took place in 2015. I intend to expand on a discussion of these shows with further audience work for a future project. In addition to these two shows it is also worth mentioning Netflix-distributed American comedy-drama film *Private Life* (2018). This film tells the story of a middle-aged married couple who are so desperate for a genetic child that they ask a young relative to become their surrogate, using her own egg. The implantation fails and the couple continue their search for a child through the route of adoption.

These latest additions to the surrogacy TV and film cannon infer that the legal, ethical and moral complexities of the practice are evoking public interest more than ever. As this book proposes, TV programmes such as these aim to express not only the anxieties surrounding infertility and the impact of reproductive technologies, but also to reflect the changing shape of family in modern life. In their work examining five decades of family representation on TV from the 1950s–1990s, James D. Robinson and Thomas Skill (2001) claim that how families are depicted on TV is a vital indicator of such changes, arguing: 'The fictional family on television, in its many forms, has become one of our most enduring benchmarks for making both metric and qualitative assessments of how the America family is doing in the real world' (2001, 139). However, as this book asks, how well are these shows doing in illustrating such changes? How authentic are the stories being told and how is the ideology of family (and motherhood) being constructed in the texts? As TV critic Ellen E Jones asks: 'Why has TV become obsessed with surrogate mothers?' (Jones 2017). This is a question which is explored in this project.

The Changing Consumption of TV

According to statistics portal *Statista*, an estimated 1.57 billion households across the globe own at least one TV set. A growth in internet content and streaming services is also boosting daily consumption, resulting in a decline of TVs within the home. Despite this, data indicates that Americans watch the most telly, mostly cable, amounting to a countrywide average of around four-and-a-half hours a day (*Statista.com* 2019).

Lisa Taylor and Helen Wood (2008) argue that despite changes in consumption, there is still a nostalgia for TV as a medium. As they highlight when writing about the importance of TV studies, the TV is not *just* a screen, or a 'toaster with pictures' (Taylor and Wood 2008, 145), it remains important, as it is still at the heart of culture, regardless of how or where you view it. They have been (and still are) the heart of the home, a focal point, the 'hearth', replacing the stories that were once recited by the fireside (Frith 1983; Cardiff and Scannell 1993; Silverstone 1994). Despite evolving media platforms and viewing practices, TVs in the home are getting bigger. Taylor and Wood also stress that the exploration of the audience reception of TV is also just as important, despite—or because of—this evolving uncertainty. Furthermore, it is also vital to acknowledge televisions' (and the wider media) role is not purely cultural but performs as a conduit between the political landscape and public domain. This is necessary to consider in light of the above statistics. Simon Frith (1983) stressed in his work on social class and BBC broadcasting that the medium of television can be viewed as channel which mediates the public (politics, the state) to the private (the family, the home)—the broader world entering the domestic space through telling stories.

The body of work debating the political and cultural impact of media processes is expansive, therefore I cannot go into detail here. However, one thought to consider is John Hartley's (1999) proposition, drawing on American studies scholar George Lipsitz, that TV can be understood as 'culture articulated with politics' (1999, 24). Hartley argues that TV consumption must not be solely viewed as exploitative 'always doing something to someone, always negatively' (1999, 25) but can also be seen as an educational tool which captures and promotes historical change. Although media scholars such as Nick Couldry (2002) recognise this aspect of the positive uses of television through its ability to infiltrate private and public life, he also highlights the importance of recognising the social impacts of media power, particularly through how contemporary societies are organised.[2] George Gerbner et al. (1986) explain: 'It [television] is part and parcel of our daily life. Its drama, commercials, news and other programs bring a relatively coherent world of common images and messages into every home... television is both a shaper and stable of certain lifestyles and outlooks' (1986, 17, 23). It is this relationship between the private and the public spheres and the potential ideological impact on viewers that is of interest here. As Lynn Spigel (2005) rightly highlights: 'Who knows what audiences are seeing – much less thinking anymore? I will leave this issue to the social scientists' (in Taylor and Wood 2008, 146). This statement captures this book's central essence and emphasises the value of undertaking text and audience work, with specific attention to how the central narratives are constructed.

Narrative Analysis

Tzvetan Todorov's (1990) five stages of narrative was considered the most useful framework to employ for the narrative analysis. The narrative of a text, as argued by Seymour Chatman (1980) is the 'what' of the story, the 'way' of the narrative is the 'discourse'. As Stuart Hall argued, narrative and discourse analysis work together in a system of representation (1997). Therefore, through the application of Todorov's narrative structure: the goal, equilibrium, disruption, resolution, final equilibrium, the 'what' of the story can be illuminated, and connections with similarities and differences can be made across the texts.

In relation to this narrative structure, I have also employed Lauren Berlant's interpretation of genre as 'an aesthetic structure of affective expectation' which 'locates real life in the affective capacity to bracket many kinds of structural and historical antagonism on behalf of finding a way to connect with the feeling of belonging to a larger world, however aesthetically mediated' (2008, 4). It is her claim that women's popular culture is marked by the *femininity* of genre which is of particular applicability to this model of narrative analysis, specifically her use of the 'blockage'. For Berlant, the blockage, or surprise, is part of the convention of the femininity of genre, in the sense that it conjures the prospect of failure, and 'moments of potential collapse that threaten the contract that genre makes with the view to fulfil expectations' (2008, 4). Berlant argues that the resolution in the narrative provides a comfort in the utopia of normativity, providing a sense of belonging through the cultivation of fantasies, 'an alleviation of what is hard to manage in the lived world' (2008, 5). I will argue, based on the audience data, that there is some resistance to the blockages and resolutions embedded in the texts—a resistance to ideologies of normative heterosexuality—such as the rescuing of infertility through heterosexual love and monogamy, which emerge as central narrative conclusions across the range of genres in focus.

Genre

In addition to traditional method of textual analysis, genre analysis is also imperative to this study. Each TV show that has been selected has its own style, with its own set of codes and conventions that belong to its genre—it has its own language. As outlined by Lisa Taylor and Andrew Willis (1999): 'the acknowledgement of the genre is dependent upon an accepted set of generic conventions which enable the audience to key into the text with certain expectations' (1999, 57). These codes and conventions are constructed through the production process—from the style of filming, camera angles, close-ups, soundtrack and programme length, through to how the narrative is developed and the style of performance by the actors—all of which contribute to how emotion is constructed in the text and its ability to move audiences affectively during the viewing process (Feuer 1983; Gorton 2009; Smith 1995; Williams 1991). This ability to evoke—or in some cases, not evoke—emotions from viewers due to differing genre mechanisms is central to this study design as it relates to one of the core research questions, which asks how narratives of surrogacy are shaped through varying genre techniques, and whether these genre techniques shape the audience's perceptions of the surrogacy practice. As cognitive film theorist Noël Carroll suggests in his discussion of emotions and film, 'filmmakers have selected out the details of the scene or sequence that they think are emotively significant and thrust them, so to speak, in our faces' (in Gorton 2009, 79).

It is important to highlight here the blurring of genre boundaries. As Minna Aslama and Mervi Pantti (2006) highlight, genres are becoming more hybridised, across 'factual programming, fiction and entertainment' (2006, 171). There is also an argument to suggest that ideas about pure genre are now outdated due to the growth of hybrid genres. However, the importance of genre is still valid, even in a blended form, 'as they are still significant in how they operate within mixtures' (Mittell 2004, xii). A variety of genres have been elected for this study, and for focus, will be referred to through concise categorisations, such as reality TV, soap opera, sitcom, and Hollywood film. My interest in engaging with a wide range of genres is to explore the differences—and similarities—in how narratives of surrogacy are articulated. This study does not set out to perform an in-depth analysis on each genre category to the same intensity as other scholars in the field who have focused on one, such as reality TV (Biressi and Nunn 2005; Hill 2004; Holmes and Jermyn 2003; Murray and Ouellette 2008; Skeggs and Wood 2012). This is due to this project aiming to examine differences between genre techniques, through the construction and reception of the texts, to explore which genres have more impact on viewers over others.

Textual Analysis and Audience Reception

As mentioned, over the summer of 2015, I watched a lot of telly. Through this process, I was able to select a small number of shows to closely analyse, which was then followed by a dialogue with female audiences. This was an ongoing negotiation, the results of which have created this book. So, what exactly are these methods and why have I selected them to work together?

Textual analysis is a method of data analysis that closely examines either the content and meaning of texts. These texts include newspapers, TV programmes, radio programmes and blogs. Textual analysis allows the ability to examine how they operate, are constructed, and the ways in which meanings are produced (Given 2008). As Franklin (1990) has highlighted, popular representations have a social and cultural power. Critical discourse analyst Norman Fairclough (2003) also claims that 'texts can bring about changes in our knowledge (we can learn things from them), our beliefs, our attitudes, values and so forth' (2003, 8). However, to explore the texts selected for this book, textual analysis alone was not deemed adequate. As Fairclough has argued, effects of texts are mediated by meaning-making, which is why the audience reception of the texts, through the focus group method—details of which follow—has been an integral component to the analysis.

Although textual analysis has its limitations, the role of the analyst in the process must not be undervalued. Virginia Nightingale (1996) argued that due to the popularity of reception studies, the role of the analyst disappeared due to 'the heat' (1996, 63) being taken *off* the text and *on* to the audience. Textual analysis, therefore, is not insignificant in this study. It enables a framing that can be enhanced when combined with other methods. Only by having an audience to interpret these texts can any meanings be made, to acknowledge 'the world that exists outside of texts' (Lockyer in Given 2008, 866). This approach belongs to what has been called the 'ethnographic turn' in media studies, which has connected the fields of sociology and media, and which has produced a plethora of studies which have explored women's responses to popular TV in the context of everyday culture and class status (Ang 1985; Press 1991; Skeggs and Wood 2012; Skeggs et al. 2008; Wood and Taylor 2008; Wood 2009).

In addition to textual analysis, Helen Wood's (2009) texts-in-action method was also drawn upon for the research design. This method observes in real time what women say conversationally back to the television during the viewing process. This work provided an inspiration for my focus group design as I was curious to explore how participants would respond to the selected texts for this project. Wood observed how women 'talked back' to TV talk shows within their home environment, through the union of televised and lived environments. As she claimed, 'by looking at them [the participants] we can begin to see how the text is negotiated while it is *alive*' (2009, 109). Wood highlighted, through this method, the relationship between textuality and subjectivity, and how female viewers draw on their personal experiences through a self-reflexive response to specific genres. This approach resonated with the book's central research questions which ask how, and if, different genres articulate narratives of surrogacy differently, and how these representations reflect women's own situated experiences of living in the world. In addition to this, I also incorporated Jenny Kitzinger's (1994) game Agree/Disagree. This is where a group of participants discuss various statements and align them accordingly. I developed this game by using citations from the texts the participants watched during the earlier part of the session. For example, during a scene in *Coronation Street*, Beth Tinker, a character that found the surrogacy arrangement distasteful, delivered the line to a friend in the local pub: 'You never know what love is until you've had a kid'. This was a way to draw the participants back to the text. This triggered a telling debate with all three groups, which inspired discussions of love and the genetic bond which has shaped Chapter 5. I followed Kitzinger's example of asking participants to read out a statement in turn. As Kitzinger argues: 'the final layout of the cards is not important, it is this process of getting there which is revealing' (1994, 107).

As part of this text-audience rapport, Hall's now well-established encoding/decoding model (1973) was also deemed appropriate to integrate into the methods framework. Encoding/decoding is a theoretical audience reception model Hall constructed to identify the different ways viewers interpret mass media texts—as active, rather than passive, readers. David Morley's (2006) main critique of the model is that the construction and reception of texts are far more complex. For instance, the construction of the encoded textual meanings become blurred through the relationship between producers of the texts and conscious intention of broadcasters; and the decoding process is more influenced along the axes of comprehension/incomprehension than agreement/disagreement. However, as Morley has argued, it should not be dismissed as it still has much to offer. This text/reception model was an important moment in cultural studies, which enabled researchers in the field to 'appreciate the complexity inherent to the relationship between viewer and screen' (Gorton 2009, 20).

This was the first time in cultural theory that the role of the reader was respected—a pivotal turning point in audience research. This direction soon ignited a trend in audience studies. Hall proposed that readings of texts are polysemic, that 'meanings do not exist "equally" in the message: it has been structured in dominance although its meaning can never be fixed or "closed"' (Morley 1980, 10). Therefore, alternative meanings can be made that might not have been initially intended by the producers of the texts through the encoding process. In Hall's model, the decoding process is devised of three key reading categories: dominant-hegemonic (accepts the text's codes as natural), negotiated (partial acceptance, but resists and modifies in relation to own experiences), oppositional (understands the dominant reading but rejects it).

Despite its failings, and being over four decades old, I believe this model is still useful. The three categories (dominant-hegemonic, negotiated, oppositional) have proven to be an effective reception framework to loosely draw upon in the examination of the audience data. However, I have also noted Lisa Blackman and Valerie Walkerdine's (2001) critique of Hall's model. They claim that it lacks a closer analysis of processes of affect and emotion. They argue cognitive and rational processes have taken precedence, which resonates with Larry Grossberg's (1997) belief that affect is 'the "missing link" in the understanding of media and ideology' (in Skeggs and Wood 2012, 13). There have been debates on whether affect and cognition can coexist in one system or are separate systems (Zajonc 2000). As Misha Kavka (2008) explains: 'affect is opposed to cognition, or in the vernacular, feeling is opposed to thinking' (2008, 29). I have integrated the work on the affective *and* the cognitive processes of texts on audiences. This I justify, following Kavka, by drawing on Brian Massumi's (2002) understanding of how sense and sensation unify both sides: 'Sense itself ushers in the related but ambivalent term "sensation", reminding us that feeling has both external and internal components; a sensation can come from the way we (physically) register the world or (psychologically) registers the world's impact on us' (Kavka 2008, 29). This method corresponds with Beverley Skeggs and Helen Wood's (2011, 2012) research design for their work on audiences and reality television, through their methods of textual analysis, texts-in-action, focus groups and interviews, a framework that has helped shape the design for this project. I too am concerned with 'audience encounters and interactions with the television through empirical research' (Skeggs and Wood 2012, 136).

Charlotte Brunsdon and David Morley (1978) applied the encoding/decoding model to *The Nationwide Project*—an ethnographic experiment on audiences in London and the Midlands. Morley later continued this work in his own project, *The Nationwide Audience* (1980). One main criticism he expressed of his own research design was that selecting the texts for the audiences was artificial. However, in relation to this project, where I have also selected the texts for the viewing sessions, I believe this is not a core concern, due to the nicheness of the subject matter—very few of the participants were familiar with the surrogacy narratives.

In addition, a preselection of the material was necessary to ensure structured viewing in light of contemporary reception frames, which includes, for example, viewing multiple screens in public spaces, the viewing of texts on portable electronic media, and enhanced viewer control through remote control channel-flicking (Ang 1991, 1995; Bellamy and Walker 1996; McCarthy 2001; Uricchio 2005). Anna McCarthy (2001) calls this dislocated form of audience-text interaction 'ambient' television watching, which she argues causes fragmented concentration. Therefore, the focus group setting with supplied texts was deemed vital, to keep the participants focussed and to create a dedicated space to allow their voices to be heard.

The Focus Group—Why Listening to Women's Voices Matter

Due to the reproductive nature of surrogacy, which encompasses themes of infertility, motherhood, sexuality and family, a feminist methodological approach was elected to make women's knowledge valid and authoritative—and which puts gender as central. Janet Holland and Caroline Ramazanoglu (2002) emphasise that feminist social research gives insights into gendered social existence. Although such an approach leaves the methodology open to critiques of essentialism, the adoption of Donna Haraway's (1988) 'situated knowledges' deflects such claims. Through this concept, partial perspectives of different communities of women and their varied experiences of the world are valued. Knowledge, as Haraway argues, is an instrument of vision. It is this vision through women's interpretation of television texts which is of core value to this project.

Sue Wilkinson (1999) argues that feminist methods should be contextual, and the gathering of women's voices—and listening to them—shows a commitment to feminist research. Therefore, as women's voices are central to this project, working in dialogue with textual analysis, the focus group method was deemed appropriate as it enables a space where participants can share with the researcher, and with each other, their own experiences in relation to a specific topic (Brennen 2012; Dimitriadis and Kamberelis 2008; Wilkinson 2004). Kitzinger (2004), who researches the audience reception of social, health and scientific issues, argues that the focus group is a research tool that can help explore how media representations might relate to, and potentially influence, the public understanding of certain issues: in this project issues surrounding reproductive technology, family and motherhood.

In her work on mothers' interpretations of popular maternal representations on TV, Rebecca Feasey (2015) rightly highlights concern over the focus group setting, as some voices may dominate over others. This usually occurs in groups where the participants don't know each other, assembled through random sampling. Feasey suggests that the self-selecting of groups (work, family, social activities) within a domestic setting ensures a more relaxed and natural discussion. This I took into consideration. However, the sensitivity of the topic influenced the recruitment.

The three focus groups consisted of a total of nineteen women—mixed mothers, non-mothers and pre-mothers. The participants were aged between 17 and 43, were of differing sexual identities and came from varying professional, cultural and class backgrounds. Some were single, some married. Some didn't want kids, some did—some couldn't. The mixed mothers group is described as mixed as it included non-mothers, mothers and pre-mothers. The non-mothers group consisted of women who didn't want children and those who were unsure about having children. The pre-mothers group consisted of young teenage women at a different life stage than the other participants. The motivation for these groupings was that the participants could draw on a range of positions in relation to fertility and motherhood, as they all had different experiences. It is important to emphasise here that the description 'pre-mother' is not employed with the assumption that the women are to become mothers in the future, but is a term used to frame the group in relation to their current position to motherhood, as younger women. Therefore pre-mother, in this context, is flexible, used to describe a position of non-motherhood which has the potential to change.

All the participants in the mixed mothers and non-mothers groups were known to me. They all knew about my problematic fertility background, and I knew about theirs—if they had one. I also knew about their personal relationship status, which must also be recognised as a contributory factor to non-motherhood. The mixed mothers all knew each other, either through a pre-existing mutual friendship group or having met through a previous session I had run which explored similar themes. As this group were familiar with each other, I decided to hold the session at my home. The non-mothers group didn't know each other, so I decided to hold the session within the neutral space of a room at Goldsmiths, University of London, in South East London, where this research was undertaken. I didn't know the pre-mothers sixth form school group, but they were all familiar with each other as they were in the same cohort.

It could be queried why I didn't recruit solely participants with some experience of surrogacy, and/or infertility and IVF, due to the surrogacy and infertility narratives that are central to the texts under analysis. I didn't feel this was necessary as the primary focus was to include participants with different relationships to and experiences of motherhood. However, it is important to highlight that some of the participants across the groups did have experiences of limited fertility. This was private information only known to me, and not shared with the other participants.

It is necessary to acknowledge the small size of the study sample. Bigger research projects such as Kitzinger's (1994) AIDS Media Research project undertook 52 focus group sessions, with 351 participants. Kitzinger claimed that this was necessary for the project, due to a wide focus on social context. Such an extensive use of focus groups was not necessary for this study, due to its narrow focus. However, in relation to arguments of validity due to working with a small sample, I recognise that there are limitations to these findings. For instance, the participants were all based in London, during a specific time period (twenty-first century), and within a community of English-speaking professionals. Therefore, this study is subsequently reflective of some women's experience which cannot be globalised. However, other gender and media focused research projects have also relied on small study groups. For example, Linda Duits and Pauline van Romondt Vis (2009) worked with a small group of Dutch girls aged 12–13 to investigate how young girls make meaning from celebrities. Rebecca Coleman (2008, 2012) worked with girls aged 13–14 from two schools in South London and Oxfordshire, to explore the relationship between their bodies and images. These projects, like this one, probe into the cultural zeitgeist through empirical work to explore how meanings are made and received and what this implies ideologically for not just women in modern life but those who are positioned as non-normative.

Like all research projects, I didn't know what data would emerge. This is what makes research like this so exciting. As a feminist project, these women's voices within a dialogic textual-audience analysis have inspired the shaping of the chapters and it is listening to these voices that has informed the theoretical framework. This resulted in some surprises, particularly the employment of queer theory as an analytical lens.

Queer Theory as a Tool to Explore the Non-normative

The inclusion of queer theory as a core lens materialised quite late in the research process, while I was sifting through the focus group data, exploring a range of literature and starting to sketch out the chapters. I had already engaged with some key concepts from within this field that were applicable to the project, such as Sara Ahmed's (2010) work on happiness and happy objects, and Berlant's (2011) cruel optimism—concepts that are explained in the following chapter. However, it became clear that this was a field that I could benefit from engaging with on a much deeper level.

Before I started writing up the research, I read Radclyffe Hall's (1928/2014) lesbian novel *The Well of Loneliness* and Adrienne Rich's (1980) *Compulsory Heterosexuality and Lesbian Existence*, which Ahmed discusses in her work. This was when I was able to identify similarities between heterosexual infertility and non-motherhood with the lesbian subject position, but also to get a clearer focus on how the narratives of normative family were being shaped in the TV texts I was investigating. This was a critical moment in the research process. However, it is important to highlight here that by mobilising queer theory as a lens has enabled me to explore and expose the inherent heteronormativity that I believe structures the narratives in *all* of the texts under analysis, even those featuring same-sex families that are presented as alternative.

Furthermore, as discussed throughout the book, I have also attempted to transcend hetero/homo divisions by identifying similarities on both sides of the binary. Through political scientist Cathy J. Cohen's (1997) core arguments I propose that heterosexual subjects are also regulated and excluded by dominant heterosexual culture, in the context of infertility, voluntary childlessness, and to some extent women who work as commercial surrogates. I will argue that through these representations, and through the participants own experiences, these heterosexual subject positions are also located on the fringes of the normative which might, as highlighted by Annette Schlichter (2004) 'allow for a critical analysis of his or her compliance to the dominant structure' (2004, 546).

The queer lens helps to unpick the main narrative themes in the texts, which are overwhelmingly shaped by heteronormative family bonded through romantic love and the genetic tie—the correct picture. This, as pointed out by a number of queer theorists, upholds the notion that heterosexual reproduction, monogamy and domesticity is the normative ideal that must be aspired to for subjects to belong in the world, and to *not* be categorised as deviant (Ahmed 2010; Berlant 2008; Edelman 2004; Halberstam 2011; Warner 1999). As argued by straight queer theorist Calvin Thomas (2000), there is a lot in queer theory that we straights can identify, given 'surprised perplexity at recognizing [our] own reflections in queer theory's mirror' (2000, 2).

As a heterosexual woman who experienced many years of fertility issues, I too recognise my reflection in this work. I am able to identify with the discussion of queer identities in the reflection of heteronorms. I share feelings of not fitting in, of being on the outside. Like some of the focus group participants, I too am unable to identify or relate to mainstream cultural representations of family and dominant ideologies of femininity, which convey very specific ideas of what it means to be a *real* woman. It is the elasticity of the term 'queer' that has enabled me to explore a range of identities in the reflection of familial norms that are positioned as non-normative.

It is important to emphasise here, referring to Michael Warner (1993), that the term *queer* is not about defining identities against the heterosexual, but against the heteronormative, which he proposes are two different things. It is this definition, and use of the verb term *to queer*, which helps navigate this project. Judith Butler (1993) and Lee Edelman (2004) in particular have called for the term to be deployed from its earlier use to question and reveal the heterosexual norms that dominate our culture.

The term 'queer' was initially a slang term for a homosexual, as a term of homophobic abuse. It was used to describe homosexuals and lesbians as not straight, not normal, not human (Ahmed 2004; Halperin 2003). It was reclaimed by New York activist group Queer Nation in the early nineties to celebrate difference as a form of political resistance to the violence and homophobia against homosexuals, ignited by the rise of AIDS and HIV in the late 1980s. As explained by queer theorist Anthony Slagle (1995): 'By using the term queer, Queer Nation diffuses the hate and tolerance associated with calling someone queer' (in Rand 2014, 4). It was also a term that was adopted to create a sense of belonging for those who have been made to feel marginalised by anyone in power. As argued by Allan Bérubé and Jeffrey Escoffier (1991) its aim was 'to bring together people who have been made to feel perverse, queer, odd, outcast, different, and deviant, and to affirm sameness by defining a common identity on the fringes' (in Rand 2014, 4).

From this activism, a new branch of critical theory emerged. 'Queer theory' was defined by feminist philosopher Teresa de Lauretis, at a conference at the University of California in 1990. De Lauretis coined the term to provide a field for scholars to 'interrogate how sexuality and other differences play a fundamental role in rhetorical practice' (Slagle in Yep 2004, 129). Lauren Berlant and Michael Warner's (1995, 1998) theory of heteronormativity is central to this project. Ahmed's (2010) concept of straightening devices to minimise signs of queerness is also fundamental, to be discussed further on. Berlant and Warner propose that dominant heterosexuality is a privileged and naturalised state, an ideal—a moral accomplishment:

> Heteronormativity is more than an ideology, or prejudice, or phobia against gays and lesbians, it is produced in almost every aspect of the forms and arrangements of social life: nationality, the state, and the law; commerce; medicine; and education; as well as in the conventions and affects of narrativity, romance, and other protected spaces of culture. (1998, 554–555)

Queer theory as a lens has therefore been employed in this book to explore notions of the non-normative and the normative that have materialised through the cultural representations of surrogacy on TV and film, which, as will be discussed, revolve around narratives of romance and conventions of family. Queer theory as a lens has enabled me to expose an embedded heterosexism that I believe has been constructed in the texts. The non-normative, in the context of this study, emerges in the construction of the infertile heterosexual female characters. In addition, this theory of normativity has also informed further discussion on what is deemed acceptable and non-acceptable—normative and non-normative—in relation to the representations of lesbians, homosexuals, and people of colour.

Engaging with queer theory has also exposed the heteronorms that are constructed in the articulations of both heterosexual and homosexual couplings in relation to building families through surrogacy. This further exposes the value attached to the reproduction of white families created through heterosexual love and the genetic tie. As Alexander Doty (1993) has identified: 'within cultural production and reception, queer erotics are already part of culture's erotic centre, both as a necessary construct by which to define the heterosexual and the straight (as "not queer")' (1993, 4). Queer theory can also provide a tool to explore 'a wide range of impulses and cultural expressions, including space for describing and expressing bisexual, transsexual, and straight queerness' (1993, 2).

What I describe as a heterosexual *straight queerness* has emerged as a particular focus for this study, in relation to the representation of heterosexual female infertility and childlessness that is explored in Chapter 4. In this chapter, themes of shame, deviancy and alienation have been identified through textual analysis and audience reception. However, a homosexual *queer straightness* has also been identified in the representation of homosexuality and lesbianism, which will be discussed in Chapter 3. Drawing on Ahmed (2010), *queer straightness* is a normalising process that is shaped in the text's narratives and character constructions and positioning, through the employment of straightening devices, such as normative ideals of family, genetically related children, and monogamous relationships. As argued by Ahmed, such devices situate the characters in 'approximation to signs of straightness' (2010, 15). Therefore, a range of work within queer theory has been mobilised to explore what I will argue are problematic representations of homosexuality and lesbianism, with specific focus on how signs of queerness are minimised through the construction of heteronormativity in the texts' narratives.

Queer readings of mass culture texts, which include both straight and gay characters and narratives, have already been executed in some depth. These readings have explored, for example, cross-dressing in *Pee-wee's Big Adventure* (1985) and *Some Like It Hot* (1959) (Doty 1993; Slagle in Yep 2004) and closet homosexuality in *Seinfeld* (1989–1998) (Gantz in Thomas 2000); a forgetful mother and relationship-rejecting fish in *Finding Nemo* (2003) (Halberstam 2013) and connotations of lesbianism in *Laverne & Shirley* (1976–1983) and *Baby Mama* (2008) (Doty 1993; Winch 2012). I will also employ this method as part of my textual analysis in the reading of the relationship between the Kate (intended mother) and Angie (the surrogate) in *Baby Mama*, as discussed in Chapter 4.

As argued by Kath Browne and Catherine J. Nash (2010): '"Queer research" can be any form of research positioned within conceptual frameworks that highlight the instability of taken-for-granted meaning and resulting power relations' (2010, 4). Cohen (1997) has also argued that the category of heterosexuality must also be recognised in relation to being situated outside of dominant norms, as like homosexuality, she argues, heterosexual bodies are also regulated and excluded by dominant heterosexual culture.

It is important at this juncture to emphasise that my adoption of queer theory as a tool to explore representations of heterosexual infertility in this study has no intention of devaluing the important work queer theory and queer activism has done to challenge inequalities that exist within mainstream heterosexual culture. Through this project I also aim to challenge what Thomas (2000) has described as the 'countless reels of mainstream film and hours of compulsory heterosexual television, that gays and lesbians have suffered through the years without finding any such specific and positive trace of recognition' (2000, 19). However, in addition to this, I will propose that similarities can be drawn between what I have named the *straight queerness* of heterosexual infertility and lesbianism, as I believe these subject positions are both marginalised through popular cultural representations and can find a common identity through being situated outside of the normative.

Despite his scepticism, David Halperin (2003) argues that queer theory as a field only has future potential if new ways are found to invigorate its potential, and not through 'devising some new and more avant-garde theoretical formulation of it but, quite concretely, reinventing its capacity to startle, to surprise, to help us think what has not yet been thought' (2003, 343). Therefore, to employ queer theory as a tool to queer straight research of TV shows with surrogacy storylines must be seen as contributing to an advancement of the field.[3]

Berlant and Warner (1995, 1998) were at the forefront of recognising cultural and political fixation with normativity, and the importance of holding a queer lens over popular culture to expose heterosexism. As they claim: 'It is no accident that queer commentary – on mass media, on texts of all kinds, on discourse from science to camp – has emerged at a time when United States culture increasingly fetishizes the normal' (1998, 345). As Thomas (2000) highlighted, there is a lot in queer theory for us straights to get excited about.

The Perpetuation of the White American Dream—On and Off TV

Michèle Barrett and Mary McIntosh (1991) argued for the importance of analysing cultural texts within the historical context of the time. Therefore, it is imperative to acknowledge the geographical location of the TV shows selected for this project. Most have been produced in America, depicting American life using American actors in American cities, apart from British soap treasure, *Coronation Street* and the Australian made *Top of the Lake: China Girl*. Due to its arrival post-research, the latter is reflected upon throughout the book in relation to core themes that have been identified, but not fully explored.

The differences in how *Corrie* emotionally connected with the focus group participants compared to the American shows are explored in Chapter 2. As will transpire throughout the book, this domination is significant content-wise, particularly in light of how (and why) the white, heterosexual normative family is not only shaped in mainstream American culture, but championed through forceful political agendas in a present-day America that oppress those who wish to live comfortably outside (or inside) the white picket fence: immigrants, single mothers, gays, the disabled, and those of colour.

The shows under analysis all infer that the ideal American family is white. This value of whiteness is explored throughout the chapters. One critical example is the construction of the black characters in *The New Normal* (Rocky) and *Baby Mama* (Oscar) which as I argue are inserted into the narrative to support white sentimentality by helping to keep white families together through subservient positioning, as discussed in Chapter 4. I believe this reflects traces of the mammy film stereotype of the 1930s; instrumental figures who maintained the white happy household (Bogle 2016). In addition to this, the research findings also reveal that a primary theme is that reproductive technologies are only made available to a specific type of user, one who is white, heterosexual, married and middle class. With this in mind, it is imperative to acknowledge the sociopolitical context within which these programmes were made. Therefore, key events *outside* of the television screen are important to mention.

Berlant (2008) argues that America is a country dedicated to reproducing the normative, an aspiration organised through convention which gives its citizens power through the fantasy of belonging. Laura Briggs (2017) claims that the fertility industry in America is steered by the eugenics movement and fuelled by the politics of racial division. Trump's unashamed racist rhetoric throughout his campaign and time in office is clearly indicative of this. Real-world incidents outside of these surrogacy storylines can help demonstrate the racially skewed reproductive politics in America. The rescue effort in New Orleans after Hurricane Katrina hit in 2005 is a good example. According to a range of news reports, Louisiana's governor Kathleen Bianco authorised the rescue of stored frozen embryos from a fertility clinic based in Lakeside hospital in eastern New Orleans while the city was in lockdown. State troopers, doctors and trucks were mobilised to save these future white children. A number of stories about these 'earliest survivors' (Goldenberg 2017) later emerged in the mainstream media, white children hailed as miracles born from devastating circumstances. However, the media also reported that while these embryos were being saved, black residents were left to die. As New Orleans, racial justice spokesperson Latoya Lewis claims: 'Katrina was one of the most modern times where this country showed us how they feel about black people and people of color' (Finley 2015).

So, if the majority of the TV shows are American, why base the audience research in Britain, with mainly British participants? As has been discussed, TV and media content are distributed and accessed globally. A range of TV programs circulate through the unrelenting surge of on-demand, online and cable content. It is how this content is able to flow universally with such ease that is a central motive for this study—specifically in relation to the dissemination of a normative family ideology which upholds the white, heterosexual family as the ideal and firmly positions women in a normative role as wives and mothers. Therefore, despite the TV shows examined in this book being predominantly American, and the location of the focus groups being in Britain, the findings have produced important and valuable insights. Like media scholar Andrea Press (1991) who explored women's responses to TV's portrayal of the nuclear family, I am also concerned with how television influences women's identities in their wider cultural environment, principally in the context of not just the whitewashing of the ideal family structure, but what have been identified as archaic notions of motherhood, family, femininity and sexuality.

Family Ideology and Its Circulation on TV

Radical feminist Shulamith Firestone (1970) argued that the biological family must be dismantled; women liberated from reproduction for true emancipation. In contrast to this belief, Barrett (1984) and Barrett and McIntosh (1991) claim that despite the demise of the nuclear model, the family still maintains a popular appeal, which is reproduced through willing participants. As they argue in their work on the ideology of family in advanced capitalist societies, the image of the family in modern life still depends on this 'combination of the natural and the moral' (1991, 27). They propose that this construction of the normative family ideal, as pictured through nineteenth-century notions of motherhood within the breadwinner family and the home as haven (Lasch 1991) is entrenched in the ideological structuring of contemporary society, indicative of an ideology of family that moves beyond the narrow definitions of the economic unit.

However, what Barrett and McIntosh are able to identify in more modern social contexts is how ideals of family exist, for instance, in school curriculums, advertising campaigns and holiday brochures. Barrett (1991) claims Stuart Hall's (1973) theory of representation is useful to consider in the examination of how the ideology of family is *represented* and culturally *reproduced* through the cultural products of TV and film. Furthermore, Barrett argues the cultural reproduction of family ideals is an important development, a crucial dimension that requires scholarly attention. It is this form of analysis that captures, more accurately, the work of ideology within historical conditions, but positions the subject as an active participant rather than a passive consumer.

Barrett and McIntosh identify the importance of how family ideology is constructed through television texts, specifically within the soap opera genre through the work of Charlotte Brunsdon (1997). They cite Brunsdon's work on Britain's *Crossroads* as a core example of how the family must be analysed as anything other than private, as familialism 'pervades not merely women's soap opera but virtually every cultural genre' (in Barrett and McIntosh 1991, 130). Hamid Naficy (1989) also stresses that television reproduces the nuclear family as a leading social kinship model, despite its fragmentation. Stephanie Coontz (1993) proposes that the most prevailing picture of traditional families in America 'derive from images that are delivered into our homes in countless reruns of 1950s television sit-coms' (1993, 23). In relation to motherhood, Feasey (2013, 2015) highlights that popular media texts construct, circulate and conform to ideologies of mothering 'through parenting manuals, mainstream film, news reports, advice columns, women's magazines, celebrity-led publications, and adver-tising' (2015, 2). She also emphasises the importance of examining and challenging the depictions of motherhood on TV, as representations under the entertainment category should be taken seriously, particularly through how they address female viewers.

However, although emphasising the importance of the cultural constructions of family and motherhood in popular culture, what has been predominantly overlooked, and which I attempt to expose throughout this project, is the call for a closer examination of the popular cultural articulation of the ideology of romance through not only notions of conventional femininity, which as I argue reproduce and maintain normative family, but a shift in the romance narrative. As I have identified across all the texts in focus, the search for romantic love has been replaced with the search for a child—romance to follow—through what Rosalind Gill and Elena Herdieckerhoff (2006) have called a *rewriting* of romance. They claim that writers have revised traditional romance novels for new audiences, which has created new subgenres of women's literature, such as chick lit. Applying the idea of the rewrite to film and TV texts, I argue that in contrast to the 'pregnancy first, romance after' narrative of the mom-com (Oliver 2012), the vehicle for romance in *Baby Mama* is the desire for the *future foetus*. The *future foetus* in this project describes the embryo that's yet to be formed; the child that's yet to be conceived. This desire can be described through what I call the delayed conception plotline. This is an extension of the 'delayed consummation plotline' (Scodari in Battles and Hilton-Morrow 2002, 92), where the interaction of characters in the narrative is driven by the search for a romantic relationship. In my expansion, the narrative focus is on the search for the *future foetus*, and not the male partner—the primary goal being to achieve motherhood status, through natural pregnancy or surrogacy.

Berlant claims that the heterosexual love plot creates a fantasy world which women 'experience affectively without being able to live it objectively' (2008, 31), institutions of heterosexual love enabling the possibility of a path to a better life, through the notion of rescue. As she argues: 'To be needed (by a lover, children, a family, or all of them, in a nimbus of intimate connections) demonstrates your feminine worth'

(2008, 171). Once again, maternal femininities are indicative of fulfilment rather than duty (Baraitser and Tyler 2010; Kaplan 1992). Furthermore, Berlant also suggests that to live affectively in a sentimental fantasy world is pleasurable for female audiences, as it enables feelings of belonging to a larger world. Janice Radway's (1983, 2) seminal work on the romance novel also proposes that women use the romance fiction genre to escape from the drudgery, sadness and disappointment of their daily lives, and to identify with a heroine who has a better life. Radway argues through her empirical work with romance readers that audiences respond positively to independent heroines, which highlights 'patriarchal marriage's failure to address their needs' (1983, 68). However, despite this, she discovered her participants found most pleasure in conventional narratives, where the heroine ends up rescued by a man. In this research project, I have encountered the opposite. The audience data in my sample revealed desires to see more unconventional endings that didn't default to this outmoded narrative. This is discussed in Chapter 5.

Despite this, overall, romance sells. Berlant highlights that women's culture (films, fiction, etc.) is a lucrative industry that targets women for profit, capitalist culture influencing emotional lives, which I call a capitalisation of *womanhood*. Through this rewriting of the romance narrative—where the *future foetus* is the goal, and not the romantic partner—Berlant's notion of rescue is particularly useful to extend, as it performs as a vehicle to restore norms outside of the conventional boy-meets-girl narrative. In addition, Oliver's (2012) work on how female characters in Hollywood films are transformed through pregnancy, or in Oliver's argument, 'domesticated' or 'tamed' (2012, 61, 67) is also useful to evoke for this discussion. I will argue, drawing on the audience data that highlights how the narrative closures in the texts all adhere to convention, that the female characters in the texts are repositioned within the domestic space, as mothers. This echoes the figure of the nineteenth-century mother who has been repackaged through the notion of postfeminist domestic pleasure (Gill 2007; Gill and Herdieckerhoff 2006[7]; McRobbie 2004) and returned through the restoration narrative. As Janet Walker (1982) explains in her discussion of Hollywood films that feature strong female characters: 'Often narrative closure itself seems to necessitate the resolution of problems and ambiguities brought up by the desire of women characters to go to work, to be sexual beings, or both. The end of the story becomes the solution of that story when the woman is returned to her "proper" place, i.e., with her husband, at home' (1982, 167). A successful career is not enough, whereas fulfilment through pregnancy and motherhood *is* (Kaplan 1992; Oliver 2012; Winch 2012[1]). This is explored in Chapter 4 through the discussion of the characters Kate in *Baby Mama* and Audrey in *Rules of Engagement* who both put their careers ahead of having a child, which as the narrative indicates, has affected their fertility. Both characters magically get pregnant through normative heterosexual sex, which as I argue repositions them within the home into a normative female.

I will argue that this 'renewed sentimentalizing motherhood discourse' (Kaplan 1992, 195) gains cultural currency by protecting the collapse of the nuclear family from infertility and the threat of childless women. Furthermore, in an extension of the restoration narrative, I also argue how homosexual parents-in-waiting are also 'tamed'. This is tackled in Chapter 3, where I propose the homosexual male characters are restored to the normative in the reflection of the nuclear family model, to make homosexuality and same-sex parenting more palatable to mainstream audiences. In his discussion of gay parenting in *The New Normal* and *Modern Family*, André Cavalcante (2014) argues that while offering a new family form to audiences, the gay characters in these shows have to be domesticated and like heterosexuals 'to embody dominant conceptions of social worth and legitimacy', engaging with 'textual strategies that make them more agreeable or "normal" to viewers who might feel troubled by their presence' (2014, 460).

Furthermore, in the case of *Baby Mama* and *Rules of Engagement* as explored in Chapter 5, the power of heterosexual sex through romantic love conquers technology as the cure for childlessness (see also Oliver 2012) which not only rescues the infertile woman from the shame of infertility, to make her complete as a woman—but also rescues the *future foetus*. In addition, it will also be suggested that it is not solely heterosexual love that rescues the infertile women, and which reproduces the future family, but it is the *future foetus* that swoops in to save the day. Instead of being progressive—which these surrogacy storylines initially indicate—I will argue that the family ideologies that penetrate the contemporary texts under analysis are in fact regressive, in the sense that nineteenth century ideals of monogamy, heterosexuality and domesticity are reiterated through the cultural reproduction of the family on TV. However, in addition to the shift in the romance narrative, what has also been identified is how broader narratives of family ideology have been culturally cultivated on and off our TV screens, from early foetal imaging to the fetishisation of the pregnant female body.

Foetal Attraction—From the Sonogram to Demi Moore

Franklin (1991) argues that the emergence of science and visualisation technologies were fundamental to the shaping of foetal personhood, primarily through the spectacular imagery that was made visible through the development of the ultrasound. Kelly Oliver (1997) argues that foetal personhood materialised when the foetus was no longer regarded as a collection of cells and tissue, but a small person. This emerged through not just the development of ultrasound scans, but practices of genetic testing and nutritional practices. Cynthia Daniel (2009) and Sara Dubow (2011) have emphasised the importance of the transition from foetal personhood to foetal citizen through their exploration of state power and foetal rights in America. Both argue that through the foetus being viewed as a little person in utero, it came to be viewed as vulnerable, with rights, that needed state protection. Oliver (1997) highlights how this shift in power repositioned the mother as a threat, as someone who 'becomes suspect and responsible for any defects, both physical and psychological, in the child' (1997, 27).

The framing of the foetus as a helpless victim to be saved from the danger of its mother (or hosting body, such as a surrogate) evoked wide feminist and philosophical debates, particularly through medical and legal intervention, as not all future citizens are wanted, by pregnant women or by the state. This has been explored through discussions on foetal rights and abortion (Berlant 1994; Johnsen 1986; Oaks 2000; Petchesky 1987; Katz Rothman 2000), the biological threat of women of colour (Roberts 2014) and maternal neglect through drug abuse (Beckett 1995; Boudreaux and Thompson 2015; DeVille and Kopelman 1998; Flavin and Paltrow 2010; Lester et al. 2004; Losco 1989).

Daniel (2009) and Dubow (2011) claim that the state required the *future foetus* to be protected (white) or stopped (non-white) *before* conception, through prenatal healthcare, government intervention on family planning and the distribution of contraception. While the American pro-life agenda during this period intended to save the *future foetus* (as it still does now), black women's bodies were being targeted to prevent them, through enforced sterilisation.[4] Roberts (2000) claims this eugenics programme began during the mid-twentieth century, targeting those who were deemed less valuable in society, such as poor women and women of colour. The Black Nationalist movement fought against this prevention for racial progress (Nelson 2003; Treadwell 1972).

Joanne Finkelstein (1990) and Angela Davis (1983; Davies 1998) propose that the cult of motherhood in the nineteenth century has re-emerged in contemporary attitudes to reproductive technologies. In her discussion of the high cost of the assisted reproduction industry in America, Laura Briggs (2017) also claims that reproductive technologies are steered by the eugenics movement, its aim to enable the white professional class to reproduce. In addition, Finkelstein also argues that modern medicine aims to restore infertile women to her 'natural condition, that of a child-bearer' (1990, 14) which she believes reflects the nineteenth-century belief that biology is destiny.

This book extends these debates by examining the cultural construction of the female subject's *desire* for the *future foetus*, through a baby hunger (Davitz 1984; Hewlett 2002; Kaplan 1992). This builds on Petchesky's (1987) discussion of how anti-abortion propaganda shows foetal images being saved that are 'younger and younger, and tinier and tinier… the point of vulnerability being "pushed back" *indefinitely*' (1987, 272). I will argue that this vulnerability is being pushed back even further, through the fear of losing the foetus prior to conception. Here it is not just the maternal body that is considered a threat, but also the woman's infertility.

Although this book is not exploring foetal representations, the *future foetus* is taking centre stage as *getting* the foetus (and then the baby) through surrogacy drives the narratives across the texts. This shows how cultural representations have shifted from looking inside the body (foetal imaging) to the foetus then being re-enveloped back inside the body (pregnancy)—which is discussed further on—to what I will argue is a new phase of cultural work that focuses on the *future foetus*.

Fears of infertility and loss of the *future foetus* are constructed in the texts as the fear of *no future*—or in this context, *no foetus*. Edelman (2004) has argued that this fear of *no future*, which describes the anxiety of a future void of the child, is associated with homosexual sex for pleasure, rather than procreation. Edelman claims that homosexuals are considered a reproductive threat to the future as well as feminists and pro-abortionists. I extend this in Chapter 4 by including the infertile. Here I will develop the notion that the foetus needs rescuing from the hostility of the woman's body in two ways—through the monitoring of the surrogate body during gestation (the maternal body) and by the fixing of infertility through heterosexual romance. These extensions will be applied through the analysis of the surrogate characters in *Rules of*

Engagement and *The New Normal*, and the infertile characters in *Rules of Engagement* and *Baby Mama*. In the latter, both infertile characters conceive naturally through heterosexual sex. This not only completes them as a woman but rescues the *future foetus*. I also argue that such heteronormative structures further domesticate 'woman' to her 'natural' position within the home, as a mother and child-bearer, which reproduces the vision of the normative family as the ideal (Barrett 1984; Finkelstein 1990; Oliver 2012).

Foetal visualisation technologies made an impact through the science photography of Lennart Nilsson in *Life Magazine* (1965). These images presented the foetus in utero, free-floating as if in space. This marked a shift not just in technological possibilities, but in the way women's bodies were to be perceived scientifically, culturally, and philosophically. Foetal imagery influenced the erasure of maternal subjectivity—the pregnant female body construed as separate. Through visualising techniques, the image of the foetus proliferated across popular culture, gaining new status by starring in pro-life debates (Petchesky 1987), film narratives (Berlant 1994; Kaplan 1994; Oliver 2012), and car advertisements (Taylor 1992).

Berlant (1994) and Petchesky (1987, 1998) describe the foetus' entrance into popular culture through the notion of celebrity. Petchesky explores the anti-abortion documentary *The Silent Scream* (1984) as a piece of ideological propaganda constructed through cultural representation rather than medical evidence. Petchesky claims that the use of video and photographic imagery and manipulation of techniques marked a strategic shift in communicating a pro-life agenda to mass audiences, through embracing cultural trends in American politics. Berlant approaches the media representation of the foetus as a celebrity more broadly, through the lens of cultural fixation within the pro-life politics of the time, focusing on the complexities of its articulation, in political documentaries, movies, home videos and advertisements, entering the 'public sphere of "superpersonhood"' (1996, 178). One example of how Berlant unpacks these representations is illustrated in film *Look Who's Taking* (1989), through the pro-life device of the foetal diary. Anne Kaplan (1994) highlights in her analysis of these films that the foetal voice is heard and personhood is shaped at the moment of conception, 'as if he is fully cognizant from the start' (1994, 128).

As previously argued, cultural texts must be studied in relation to the historical moment. Kaplan suggests that such a representation has materialised during a period in America where 'women have won more freedoms' (1994, 11). She argues: 'How do we account for this?… Is the foetus the new savior of mankind, delivering us from the actual messes we have made? Is the focus on it part of man's dream to make the perfect being?… Focus on the foetus may, indeed, indicate a renewed desire to write the mother out of the story' (1994, 209). However, although the desire for the *future foetus* drives the narratives in the texts, in these new articulations the foetus has lost its voice by disappearing from the dual plotline, it only makes an occasional cameo appearance through the device of the ultrasound image or foetal scan, rather than taking the lead role. However, this isn't to say the foetal *presence* is not as powerful.

This foetal ideology of the white male has materialised in films such as comedy *Innerspace* (1987) where a miniature Dennis Quad (Lt. Tuck Pendleton) is accidentally shot into the butt of anxious and effeminate Martin Short (Jack Putter). Berlant (1994) points out that through this union: 'Short is masculinized and heterosexualized by carrying Quaid in his body' (1994, 190). I will extend this in Chapter 3 through the discussion of lesbian character Brenda in *Rules of Engagement* who, through her surrogate pregnancy, becomes constructed as more feminine—therefore more heterosexual—by turning into an emotional wreck.

Alongside film, the image of the foetus has been (and still is) elevated in advertising strategies to engage with a wider consumer market, to sell not only pro-life propaganda, but cars, snacks music and cosmetics (Lam 2015; Taylor 1992; Tyler 2011). As Janelle Taylor (1992) observes in her discussion of foetal images and abortion politics in the public sphere: 'Not long ago a foetus tried to sell me a car… flipping through a recent issue of Harper's magazine, I was both perplexed and disturbed to find myself confronted by a large sonogram image of a foetus, above the logo "Is something inside you telling you to buy a Volvo?"' (1992, 67). This signifies how the foetal image is being exploited to support wider capitalist industries. As Imogen Tyler (2011) argues maternity has become capitalised, selling everything from 'beauty products, pregnancy belly casts, photo shoots and foetal film… fertility treatments, eggs, foetuses and children' (Tyler 2011, 31). It is important to highlight how advances in popular culture, specifically through the construction of images in the media, influence these maternal markets. However, I propose that photographs have more cultural power over scientific visualisations. As Taylor (1992) claims, 'the denotative status of ultrasound images is not nearly as deeply rooted culturally as that of photographs (at least not yet)' (1992, 75).[5]

Although foetal ultrasound images have penetrated the frame of the family album as a 'Kodak moment' (Han 2008, 278) I will argue that the more traditional family photographs have more emotive power as kinship objects that signify family ideology (Ahmed 2010; Hirsch 1997) and which have a fetishist quality that can 'resurrect the dead or preserve lost love' (Petchesky 1987, 269). This will be explored further in the analysis of family photographs as a narrative vehicle in Chapter 2. Although this project is not focussed on photography, core moments in foetal and maternal image making (motherhood, pregnancy) in popular culture have created powerful cultural waves, which have therefore become crucial to family ideology in the context of maternal industries.

In the early nineties the image of the foetus was knocked off the mainstream stage through the image of a naked, heavily pregnant American actress Demi Moore, which adorned the cover of popular magazine *Vanity Fair* (1991). This image shot by Annie Liebovitz presented a sexual and hyper feminised visual articulation of pregnancy that, as emphasised by Tyler (2011) re-enveloped the foetus 'back inside the pregnant body' (2011, 76). The issue sold out, some grocery stores removing it from their shelves in disgust (Longhurst 2000). Tyler ascribes this new visibility to a fascination with celebrity and motherhood, where 'maternity has never been so visible, so talked about, so public' (2011, 22).

The Demi Moore image was a critical moment that marked a shift in culture. As argued by Michele Pridmore-Brown (2009), Leibovitz 'not only photographed American culture but also changed it' (2009, 81). I propose that this moment in photography created a similar impact to the publishing of Nilsson's foetal images in 1965. Like the foetus over two decades earlier, this was the first time a pregnant body had been so publicly presented. Sandra Matthews and Laura Wexler (2000) argue that this was the first time a mother (to be) was marketed as a cover girl, 'an object of the gaze packaged to create and play on the desires of the viewer' (2000, 201). Like the celebrity foetus the image of celebrity pregnancy soon became a cultural obsession, which inspired a proliferation of white sexualised images of famous pregnant female celebrities across popular media—and less famous women—reflecting similar poses. This led to the image of the pregnant female body becoming popularised on TV and on the Hollywood screen (Baraitser and Tyler 2010; Battles and Hilton-Morrow 2015; Oliver 2012; Tyler 2001, 2011).

Following Barrett's and McIntosh's (1991) work on family ideology I argue that this obsession with pregnancy images illustrates a contemporary media articulation of the nineteenth-century bourgeois ideal. Norms of family are reproduced through the elevation of white, heterosexual and *fertile* women. In this cultural ideological phase, the ideology of family comes packaged in not the cult of motherhood and the rearing of children, which Barrett and McIntosh identified as being hidden in 'the curricula of schools' and 'in the catalogues of Mothercare' (1991, 28–29), but through what I will call the cult of pregnancy. This describes the public display of the *ability* to get pregnant amassing social and cultural value, and which, as I will suggest, aims to placate anxieties of the possibility of a future void of the child (Edelman 2004; Gentile 2011).[6] Katie Gentile (2011) proposes in her work on pregnancy images in the media that such representations aim to reinforce traditional gender roles and organise culture during a time of upheaval, which I propose resonates with the cult of domesticity that arose in the nineteenth century.

The visualisation of pregnant embodiment which has eclipsed the foetus is a further reminder of the cult of motherhood and value of reproduction that situates the woman in her natural condition as a child bearer (Davis 1983, 1998; Finklestein 1990). As has been stated, clothed pregnant bodies were once viewed by popular culture with disgust and discomfort. Now, like the image of the foetus in advertising, these bodies that are driven by celebrity and consumer culture are also mobilised as a commodity, to sell commodities, the pregnant body propelled out of 'clinics, hospitals and scientific and healthcare manuals' and onto the 'catwalk, dancing in pop videos, acting in soap operas, featuring in advertising campaigns and spectacularly visible on cinema screens' (Baraitser and Tyler 2013, 7).[7]

It is important to emphasise that these critiques of the public fascination with pregnancy spotlighted here are not meant to shame the pregnant female subject, or to put forth an anti-pregnancy or maternal position, but to shed light on what I believe can and has been read as the exploitation of fertile bodies in the capitalisation of motherhood. As I will argue throughout the book, popular culture and technology *cannot* be viewed as separate entities but seen as working together in the shaping of ideologies of motherhood and family under modern capitalism. Therefore, from images of the foetus to the pregnant body, my focus now turns to images of motherhood.

The Fetishisation of the Maternal—Chav Mums and Yummy Mummies

From reproductive technologies and pregnancy being a lucrative consumer market, a new shift in the maternal industries was to follow. As Jo Littler (2013) highlights in her discussion of sexualised constructs of pregnant women—the desirable post-pregnant mother signified the shift from pregnant sexy to mother sexy, which surfaced in the trail of the Demi Moore media frenzy. A new wave of sexualisation of motherhood soon followed, primarily through the British cultural stereotype of the 'yummy mummy'. Littler claims this term describes a mother who is white, heterosexual, thirty-something, hyper-feminine, and in a position of privilege. Stephanie O'Donohoe (2006) also explores the figure of the yummy mummy in advertising, which she argues is used to sell washing powder, prams, beauty products and breastfeeding. Both scholars argue that the yummy mummy is a brand with cultural and economic currency that drives consumerism under the guise of maternal aspiration. This will be explored in Chapter 2 through the participants discussion of Giuliana in *Giuliana & Bill*.

In contrast to the yummy mummy is the British working-class single mother, described in the media as a chav mum (Littler 2013; McRobbie 2004; Skeggs and Wood 2011; Tyler 2008). This stereotype ignited moral panic within the media and right-wing government, which Beverley Skeggs (2005) argues depicted them as 'the source of all national evil' (2005, 965). Unlike the yummy mummy, these women were seen as abject, producing children at a young age unlike their yummy mummy elders who often delay motherhood due to pursuing a career (Littler 2013). Unlike the yummy mummy, the chav mum is positioned as a bad mother, portrayed as poor, lazy, cheaply dressed—symbolic of not just the failure of femininity, but a failure of *everything*. As a single mother, the chav mum is situated outside the normative picture of the proper family.

I propose this stereotype has been shaped by the media to reflect the moral panic around single mothers on welfare—much like America's welfare queen. As proposed by Briggs (2017) in her analysis of America's welfare reform, the (black) welfare queen was a type constructed by the Reagan administration in the seventies, portrayed as lazy, promiscuous and fraudulent. Briggs argues that such a character was shaped through political rhetoric to perform as a 'cover story for reducing government programmes' (2017, 47). Briggs also highlights that during Clinton's welfare reform in the nineties, the black welfare queen image of the economic parasite was still prolific, despite the majority of welfare recipients at this time being white. Once again, the narrative centres on class, status, race and notions of what makes a good mother and what are desirable future citizens—i.e. not black or mixed raced crack babies from a broken home.[8]

In the context of this project, it is also important to discuss the American equivalents of these British stereotypes—'the 'MILF' (Mother I'd Like to Fuck) and 'white trash'. This MILF evolved out of porn culture, a female archetype that is white, heterosexualised and middle class, and into younger men (Friedman 2014; Littler 2013). As May Friedman (2014) points out, the MILF's affiliation with motherhood is a relatively new twist, now reshaped as a 'naughty older mother' (Friedman 2014, 50). Tyler (2008) proposes that white trash is similar to the white chav as they both signify class disgust, 'a whiteness contaminated with poverty' (2008, 25). Tyler suggests both exhibit a contamination of whiteness through not only an appropriation of American black culture, but through the racial mixing of their children. This reflects America's racist political rhetoric of the 1960s–1980s (which still exists) that viewed black mothers as the producers of failures, black families seen as an inadequate underclass. The New Orleans rescue effort in 2005 clearly illustrates this.

This research project has revealed that white purity through the genetic tie is core to reproductive technologies (Coontz 1993; Roberts 1996; Winddance Twine 2011) and has been identified as central to the normative depictions of family. As I argue in Chapters 3 and 4, ideologies of race and class within family ideals materialise through the stereotype of white trash, which shape the characterisations of both American surrogates in *Baby Mama* (Angie) and *The New Normal* (Goldie). However, it is the construction of Angie in *Baby Mama* as white trash that engaged the focus group participants the most. When Angie is exposed as carrying her own genetic baby and not Kate's (the intended mother), Kate calls her 'ignorant white trash'. Although most of the participants found this distasteful, what this description did was to highlight how differences in relation to class and status between the surrogate and the intended mother has been shaped in the narrative. This is examined in Chapter 4. In addition, I will also argue that the figure of the MILF can be identified in the depiction of the American intended mothers.

This is explored, in the same chapter, in the discussion of Kate's makeover scenes in *Baby Mama*.

I argue these portrayals demonstrate that heterosexual pairing and the value of perpetuating the genetic bond are also shaped by class differences, which aim to infer social and cultural notions of what makes a mother good, or bad. I also discuss how good and bad motherhood is also depicted through stereotypical representations of race and sexuality. For example, although the focus group participants did not directly discuss race in relation to motherhood, what they did was to identify how black characters are often not assigned lead roles but are constructed in such a way as to be laughed at. This is explored in Chapter 3 through the discussion of subsidiary character Rocky in *The New Normal* and the adoption storyline.

Furthermore, motherhood and lesbianism are also explored through the participants responses to the portrayal of lesbian surrogate character Brenda in *Rules of Engagement*. Here I argue, based on their responses, how lesbian characters must be heterosexualised for mainstream straight audiences. As Kim Akass and Janet McCabe (2006) highlight through their analysis of primetime American TV show *The L Word* (2004–2009), which follows the lives of a group of lesbians and their friends, this includes how lesbians must be placed within heteronormative narratives (in this context, pregnancy and family) and made sexually attractive to straight men. Through this discussion, I argue that lesbians are rarely represented as mothers. Furthermore, in the discussion of lesbian ambiguity that's played for a joke between the two women in *Baby Mama*, I also claim that the narrative insists that a heterosexual man must appear to restore order. Therefore, I argue in Chapter 5 that such characters emerge during a period when normative family is under threat; anxieties projected onto a woman who occupies a non-traditional role. As Kaplan argues, such figures 'represent everything that threaten the biological nuclear family' (1992, 199). As Kaplan (1992) highlights, there has been a shift. Women no longer *have* to get pregnant—they *want* to. This can be seen in the growing popularity of reproductive technologies, and in the cultural narratives of family and motherhood that are under scrutiny for this project.

Furthermore, in relation to this desire for a child, Barrett and McIntosh (1991) recognise that normative constructions of family that dominate the cultural and political landscape can also cause anxieties and insecurities. They propose that modern life should become more open to alternatives and different family formations. In the context of this project, this includes families or life choices situated outside of the idealised picture of the white heterosexual nuclear family, that are portrayed across the TV texts in question as unconventional—non-normative—in need of fixing through the help of reproductive technologies. These include same-sex and single parents, non-genetic kinship structures, and women choosing or accepting life paths outside of heterosexual monogamy and motherhood.

Fitting and Misfitting Through Reproductive Technologies

In Carla Lam's (2015) investigation into feminism and reproductive technologies, she explores the body within a material dimension, primarily through the notion that lived material realities shape how we think and structure our experiences (also see Grosz 1994). A core concept she provides for this is the reproductive misfit, which captures the tension between the (reproductive) female subject and the (social) world; flesh and environment, body and world—fitting and misfitting. Lam unpacks this dynamic by identifying and tackling scientific discourse and culture as masculine, primarily through illuminating the terms employed to describe the pregnant body as a method by which to normalise the reproductive experience for men who cannot experience reproductive labour.

This masculinisation and domination of modern technology is historically linked to patriarchy and industrial capitalism, which resonates with feminist theories of the masculinisation of the state in relation to domesticity and gender roles (MacKinnon 2000). As Constance Faulkner and Sara Weir (2004) argues, both are 'linked symbolically by themes of control and domination' (2004, 226). In addition, the state has been identified as intervening in foetal rights as a form of masculine control over women's bodies (Dubow 2011). However, as Lam points out, reproductive technologies which have enabled practices such as surrogacy have introduced a 'masculinization of motherhood' by allowing women to become fathers by receiving their child 'without labour of pregnancy or birthing' (2015, 33). This is an observation that has emerged as significant in the research in the discussion of the intended mothers' position.

Central to this materialist dimension is how foetal imaging in the 1960s, alongside the emergence of reproductive technologies, obscured the focus of the female subject, erasing maternal subjectivity and creating a loss of social, cultural and political power. As has already been discussed in detail, a wide body of work emerged during this period across Britain and America, claiming that through foetal imaging maternal subjectivity is made invisible, the pregnant body constructed as conceptually separate. It has been suggested that foetal imagery creates these boundaries by constructing the foetus as autonomous from the mother by being pictured outside of the female body.

Radical feminists in opposition to reproductive technologies mobilised science-inspired metaphors used to describe this separation, particularly in relation to the *further* erasure of maternal subjectivity in the foetal/maternal dyad through surrogacy, describing pregnant women's bodies as incubators, apparatus, foetal containers, mother machines and breeders (Corea 1985, 1988; Scutt 1990; Stanworth 1987). However, it has been claimed that the conceptual dividing of body parts through these terms, or similar, have been employed by surrogates as a method to create emotional distance from the foetus. In Tilly Teman's (2005) study of how surrogates divide their pregnant bodies into maps, she identifies how 'they distinguish between parts of the body they wish to personalize and parts they wish to distance, both cognitively and emotionally' (2005, 25).

As I will argue in the discussion of the representation of the surrogate in *Giuliana & Bill* in Chapter 2, the surrogate body as object/container is still a concept that is being mobilised, the invisibility of the pregnant body made even more apparent by being elbowed out of the frame altogether during the birthing scenes, with the hospital machinery and the intended mother now taking centre stage. The dynamic between the surrogate and Giuliana is also significant in this and the other representations, which will be discussed further through how divisions are constructed between women.

Lam sifts through the extensive body of feminist engagement with reproductive technologies by dividing the work into differing positions on the practice—resistors (radical feminists: oppressive), embracers (socialist feminists: liberators) and the equivocals (both oppressive and liberatory). Building on this framework to frame the literature, resistant feminists believe that reproductive technologies are an extension of patriarchal control, an imposed violence and male plot against women

(Corea 1985, 1988; Rich 1996; Rowland 1992; Scutt 1990; Wacjman 1991). The embracing feminists argue that biological reproduction is oppressive and that to be disentangled from the process would be liberating (De Beauvoir 1972; Firestone 1970) and that technology has the capacity to dissolve the boundaries forged through the Cartesian duality (Haraway 2010; Plant 1996). The equivocals embrace science as part of life and argue that women have the right to take control of their own reproduction through individual agency (Butler 1990; Farquhar 1996; Finkelstein 1990; Franklin and McNeil 1988; Gupta and Richters 2008; Haraway 1988; Rose 1994; Sawicki 1992). Lam also emphasises how resistant feminists view the social significance of infertility as being recent, 'because we now believe NRTs [new reproductive technologies] can "cure" infertility that we believe it must be cured' (2015, 49).

Fixing the Infertile

There are varying feminist positions on infertility and IVF. Some feminists view IVF treatment as coercive and abusive, pressuring women to conform to dominant ideologies and norms of womanhood through having children (Corea 1985, 1988; Finkelstein 1990; Hollinger 1984; Rowland 1992; Scutt 1990). Others embrace technologies as a source of empowerment (Pfeffer and Woolett 1983) or view it as a method by which to fix/repair infertility by literally constructing biology (Thompson 2005). In addition, there is a body of work that explores the failure of IVF and the experiences of infertility and childlessness *after* exiting the IVF treadmill (Murdock 1990; Throsby 2004).

Karen Throsby's (2004) explores the failure of IVF. In this work, she challenges dominant representations of childless women as being selfish and child-hating or positioned as objects of pity. I argue that similar conceptions steer the constructions of the infertile characters in all of the texts in focus. Furthermore, Throsby also objects to the social and cultural assumptions that women are defined by their reproductive capacity—the desire for children being seen as natural and inevitable. Through this position, she claims that reproductive technologies are socially shaped, normalised, able to 'fix' women's failures. In addition, Throsby also tackles issues such as race and infertility and transnational consumerism of technology, which she addresses through the ideology of normative motherhood and family. This will be debated in Chapter 6 through a discussion of the representation of transnational surrogacy in *Top of the Lake: China Girl*. I will also address the constructions of infertile characters in all of the shows in focus by exploring how female viewers make sense of them in relation to their own experiences. Normative ideologies of motherhood and family are challenged by the focus group participants who request narrative conclusions to *not* revolve around the image of the perfect white mother with her miracle pregnancy.

In her analysis of infertility news stories in the popular press, Franklin (1990) highlights how alternative users such as lesbians, homosexuals and singles are excluded from the desperate infertile couple story. This she claims underlines who is deemed fit and *unfit* for normative parenthood. As Franklin explains, the happy ending is only enabled through the intervention of technology if the user is white, married and heterosexual, and that family can only become complete, normalised, through heterosexual love. This is a narrative vehicle that has also been identified in this book, discussed in relation to the romance narrative rescuing the female protagonists from infertility through natural conception, or by delivering them a genetic child through surrogacy. Furthermore, alternative life choices and potential IVF users that Franklin claims are obscured by the white, heterosexual infertile couple story will be addressed further, brought back into vision through a resistance to ideals of normative family that have emerged in the audience data and discussed in Chapter 5.

Margarete Sandelowski's (1990) study of infertility is also significant in the context of both Throsby's and Franklin's work as she addresses fictional representations of infertility in relation to the lived experiences of infertile women. Sandelowski focuses on the voids that have emerged between fertile and infertile women through categories and labelling, which she argues have been shaped through a culture that 'promotes motherhood and subverts sisterhood' (1990, 34). Sandelowski proposes that the tensions between women are not only evident in the findings in her qualitative data but endorsed in the fictional articulations of infertility in novels, which she proposes are divisive through creating difference, the result being a threat to female friendship. As she states: 'Labels such as "mother" and "infertile woman", in addition to describing women, also prescribe certain patriarchal standards and expectations for women that defy female unity' (1990, 34).

What she describes as an 'imperilled sisterhood' (1990, 33) has materialised as a dominant theme throughout all of the TV texts examined in this book, most significantly through the portrayal of the relationships between the infertile (intended mother) and the fertile (surrogate) characters. As explored in Chapter 4, the baby shower scene in *Rules of Engagement* is just one example of this. In this scene, the infertile character is excluded from the celebrations and pictured as unhappy, the surrogate the centre of attention. Sandelowski's work with women has revealed how rituals such as the baby shower ceremony make infertile women feel excluded. This construction of exclusion was detected and discussed in the audience data. Therefore, following Sandelowski, I will employ the notion of 'imperilled sisterhood' to examine how alienation and exclusion steers all of the narratives in focus. Furthermore, I will argue that such representations validate divisions between women, which are deeply entrenched in our culture.

Due to the empirical data that co-drives this project, it is imperative to acknowledge that no truth claims are made in this book. It must be emphasised that the analysis, of both the audiences and by me, the researcher, should be understood as interpretation. To make this interpretation transparent, and to invite further analysis from scholars who I hope will be inspired to build on and contribute to this area of research, substantial sections of the orthographical transcriptions have been embedded throughout the analytical chapters, which now follow.

Notes

1. Although the storyline does not precisely illustrate surrogacy arrangements due to the handmaids being forcibly impregnated and delivering babies that they—and not the intended parents—are genetically related to (most of the men are infertile), this text is still considered relevant due to the overall themes that shape the narrative.
2. It is significant to point out here recent political incidences where TV consumption has influenced politics, which demonstrates a reversal. The obvious example is Trump's election to president in 2016. It is conceivable to argue that his role on *The Apprentice* (NBC, 2004–2017) and *The Celebrity Apprentice* (NBC, 2008–2017) was the platform that helped propel him into office. Through surveying a sample of American voters, Shira Gabriel et al. (2018) concur, claiming that years of exposure to Trump on these shows formed parasocial bonds with viewers, making him familiar, real and important. This may have 'led to a predisposition to believe positive information about Trump, discount negative information, and view Trump as a good potential president' (Shira et al. 2018. 'From Apprentice

to President: The Role of Parasocial Connection in the Election of Donald Trump'. *Social Psychological and Personality Science* 9 [3]: 300).

3. This is particularly significant in light of the current rise of xenophobia that has emerged in the rhetoric of both Brexit and Trump campaigns. It is also important to note, in light of this, that the majority of the shows in focus have been produced in America.
4. It is important to note that it is not just black women's bodies that have been intruded upon by state intervention—for a comprehensive discussion on forced abortion in China due the one child policy, see Nie Jing-Bao, *Behind the Silence: Chinese Voices on Abortion* (Lanham, MD: Rowman & Littlefield, 2005).
5. Taylor rightly notes here that ultrasound images will become more advanced over time. Since her time of writing 3D and 4D scans are now available, which provide real-time development of the foetus which can be recorded and uploaded into a DVD, to be played on mobile devices or at home, which 'enables you to watch all the action in the comfort of your own home, or share on your mobile device, whether they're yawning, smiling or sucking their thumb'. Google, "Thelondonultrasoundcentre.co.uk."
6. Although not for detailed discussion here, the trend in the Hollywood inspired blue-line moments and the fast-growing online community of home birth videos are certainly indicative of this public display of value attached to fertility.
7. The image of a heavily pregnant celebrity still has massive cultural impact, but across more contemporary platforms. Where Demi Moore graced the cover of *Vanity Fair* in 1991, which boosted magazine sales and subscriptions, R&B singer Beyoncé's pregnancy image posted on Instagram in February 2017 was the most liked image on the social media platform in its history at that time, having chalked up over 11 million likes. During the final edit of this book in 2019, Kylie Jenner's image of her baby girl Stormi Webster grasping her perfectly manicured finger is at almost 19 million. This was then followed by World Record Egg's image of an uncracked egg which set out to beat Jenner's record, which they did with just over 51 million. This is fascinating in light of this book's discussion of the *future foetus*. Leibovitz, Annie, *More Demi Moore* 1991, Vanity Fair. Beyoncé, "We have been blessed." Jenner, "Stormi Webster." World Record Egg, "Let's set a world record."
8. In her work on class and gender Skeggs highlights how such conceptions around the welfare mother and crack babies in America have been recycled in Britain to describe working class single mothers as being a threat to the social order, through Conservative party politics in the mid-nineties. Beverley Skeggs, *Formations of Class and Gender: Becoming Respectable* (London: Sage, 1997).

References

Ahmed, Sara. 2004. *The Cultural Politics of Emotion*. London: Routledge.

Ahmed, Sara. 2010. *The Promise of Happiness*. Durham: Duke University Press.

Akass, Kim, and Janet McCabe, J. 2006. *Reading the "L Word"*. London: Tauris.

Ang, Ien. 1985. *Watching Dallas: Soap Opera and the Melodramatic Imagination*. New ed. London: Routledge.

Ang, Ien. 1991. *Desperately Seeking the Audience*. London: Routledge.

Ang, Ien. 1995. *Living Room Wars*. London: Routledge.

Aslama, Minna, and Mervi Pantti. 2006. "Talking Alone: Reality TV, Emotions and Authenticity." *European Journal of Cultural Studies* 9 (2): 167–184.

Atwood, Margaret. 1985. *The Handmaid's Tale*. London: Penguin.

Baby Mama. 2008. Directed and written by Michael McCullers. Film. Universal City, CA: Universal Pictures.

Baraitser, Lisa, and Imogen Tyler. 2010. "Talking of Mothers." *Soundings: A Journal of Politics and Culture* 44 (1): 117–127.

Baraitser, Lisa, and Imogen Tyler. 2013. "Private View, Public Birth: Making Feminist Sense of the New Visual Culture of Childbirth." *Studies in the Maternal* 5 (2): 1–27. http://doi.org/10.16995/sim.18.

Barrett, Michèle. 1984. "Rethinking Women's Oppression: A Reply to Brenner and Ramas." *New Left Review* 146: 123–128.

Barrett, Michèle, and Mary McIntosh. 1991. *The Anti-Social Family*. New York: Verso.

Battles, Kathleen, and Wendy Hilton-Morrow. 2002. "Gay Characters in Conventional Spaces: Will and Grace and the Situation Comedy Genre." *Critical Studies in Media Communication* 19 (1): 87–105.

Battles, Kathleen, and Wendy Hilton-Morrow. 2015. *Sexual Identities and the Media*. New York: Routledge.

Beckett, Katherine. 1995. "Fetal Rights and 'Crack Moms': Pregnant Women in the War on Drugs." *Contemporary Drug Problems* 22 (4): 587–612. https://doi.org/10.1177/009145099502200404.

Bellamy, Robert V., and James R. Walker. 1996. *Television and the Remote Control*. New York: The Guilford Press.

Berlant, Lauren. 1994. "'America, 'Fat,' the Fetus'." *Boundary 2* 21 (3): 145–195.

Berlant, Lauren. 2008. *The Female Complaint*. Durham: Duke University Press.

Berlant, Lauren. 2011. *Cruel Optimism*. Durham: Duke University Press.

Berlant, Lauren, and Michael Warner. 1995. "What Does Queer Theory Teach Us About X?" *PMLA* 110: 343–349.

Berlant, Lauren, and Michael Warner. 1998. "Sex in Public." *Critical Inquiry* 24 (2): 547–566.

Bérubé, Allan, and Jeffrey Escoffier. 1991. "Queer/Nation: OUT/Look." *National Lesbian and Gay Quarterly* 11: 13–14.

Beyoncé. 2017. "We would like to share our love and happiness. We have been blessed two times over. We are incredibly grateful that our family will be growing by two, and we thank you for your well wishes.—The Carters." Instagram, February 1. https://www.instagram.com/p/BP-rXUGBPJa/?hl=en.

Biressi, Anita, and Heather Nunn. 2005. *Reality TV: Realism and Revelation*. New York: Wallflower Press.

Blackman, Lisa, and Valerie Walkerdine. 2001. *Mass Hysteria*. London: Macmillan.

Bogle, Donald. 2016. *Toms, Coons, Mulattoes, Mammies and Bucks: An Interpretative History of Blacks in American Films*. 5th ed. New York: Bloomsbury Academy.

Boudreaux, Michael, and John Thompson. 2015. "Maternal Rights and Substance Abuse: Gestation Without Representation." *Journal of the American Academy of Psychiatry and the Law* 43 (2): 137–140.

Brennen, Bonnie. 2012. *Qualitative Research Methods for Media Studies*. London: Routledge.

Briggs, Laura. 2017. *How All Politics Became Reproductive Politics—From Welfare Reform to Foreclosure to Trump*. Berkley: University of California Press.

Browne, Kath, and Catherine Nash. 2010. *Queer Methods and Methodologies: Intersecting Queer Theories and Social Science Research*. New York: Routledge.

Brundson, Charlotte. 1997. *Screen Tastes: Soap Opera to Satellite Dishes*. London: Routledge.

Brunsdon, Charlotte, and David Morley. 1978. *Everyday Television: Nationwide*. London: BFI Institute.

Butler, Judith. 1990. *Gender Trouble*. New York: Routledge.

Butler, Judith. 1993. *Bodies That Matter: On the Discursive Limits of Sex*. London: Routledge.

Cardiff, David, and Paddy Scannell. 1993. *A Social History of British Broadcasting: Volume One 1922–1939*. Cambridge, MA: Blackwell.

Cavalcante, André. 2014. "Anxious Displacements: The Representation of Gay Parenting on Modern Family and the New Normal and the Management of Cultural Anxiety." *Television & New Media* 1 (18): 454–471.

Chatman, Seymour. 1980. *Story and Discourse: Narrative Structure in Film and Fiction*. New York: Cornell University Press.

Cohen, Cathy J. 1997. "Punks, Bulldaggers, and Welfare Queens: The Radical Potential of Queer Politics?" *GLQ: A Journal of Lesbian and Gay Studies* 3 (4): 437–465.

Coleman, Rebecca. 2008. "The Becoming of Bodies." *Feminist Media Studies* 8 (2): 163–179.

Coleman, Rebecca. 2012. *The Becoming of Bodies: Girls, Image, Experience*. Manchester: Manchester University Press.

Collins, Nancy. 1991. "Demi's Big Moment". *Vanity Fair.*

Coontz, Stephanie. 1993. *Way We Never Were: American Families and the Nostalgia Trap*. New York: Basic Books.

Corea, Gena. 1985. *The Hidden Malpractice: How American Medicine Mistreats Women*. London: HarperCollins.

Corea, Gena. 1988. *The Mother Machine*. London: The Women's Press.

Coronation Street. 1960–present. Created by Tony Warren. TV programme. Manchester: ITV.

Coudhary, Anand Amit. 2015. "SC Suggests Ban on Commercial Surrogacy." *The Times of India*, October 15. https://timesofindia.indiatimes.com/india/SC-suggests-ban-on-commercial-surrogacy/articleshow/49365734.cms.

Couldry, Nick. 2002. *Media Rituals: A Critical Approach*. London: Routledge.

Daniels, Cynthia. 2009. *At Women's Expense: State Power and the Rise of Fetal Rights*. Cambridge, MA: Harvard University Press.

Davies, Angela. 1983. *Women, Race, Class*. New York: Ballantine Books.

Davies, Angela. 1998. "Surrogates and Outcast Mothers: Racism and Reproductive Politics in the Nineties." In *The Angela & Davis Reader*, edited by Joy James. Malden: Blackwell.

Davies, Miranda. 2017. *Babies for Sale? Transnational Surrogacy, Human Rights and the Politics of Reproduction*. London: Zed Books.

Davitz, Lois. 1984. *Baby Hunger*. 1st ed. Minneapolis: Winston Press.

De Beauvoir, Simone. 1972. *The Second Sex*. Harmondsworth: Penguin Classics.

DeVille, Kenneth, and Loretta Kopelman. 1998. "Moral and Social Issues Regarding Pregnant Women Who Use and Abuse Drugs." *Substance Abuse in Pregnancy* 25 (1): 237–254.

Devine, Bronwyn. 2017. "Our Surrogacy Laws Are Not Keeping Up with the Kardashians." *The Daily Telegraph*, August 10. https://www.dailytelegraph.com.au/rendezview/our-surrogacy-laws-are-not-keeping-up-with-the-kardashians/news-story/0607c3dc7bfadce33104ca6c4b38aff7.

Dimitriadis, Greg, and George Kamberelis. 2008. "Focus Groups: Strategic Articulations of Pedagogy, Politics and Enquiry". In *Collecting and Interpreting Qualitative Materials*, edited by Norman Denzin and Yvonna Lincoln. London: Sage.

Doty, Alexander. 1993. *Making Things Perfectly Queer: Interpreting Mass Culture*. Minneapolis: University of Minnesota Press.

Dubow, Sara. 2011. *Ourselves Born: A History of the Fetus in Modern America*. Oxford: Oxford University Press.

Duits, Linda, and Pauline van Romondt Vis. 2001. "Girls Make Sense: Girls, Celebrities and Identities." *European Journal of Cultural Studies* 12 (1): 41–58.

Edelman, Lee. 2004. *No Future: Queer Theory and the Death Drive*. Durham: Duke University Press.

Everingham, Sam. 2017. Overview of Surrogacy Options. *Families Through Surrogacy*. http://www.familiesthrusurrogacy.com/wp-content/uploads/2016/04/Overview-of-Surrogacy-Options.pdf. Accessed 2 September 2017.

Fairclough, Norman. 2003. *Analysing Discourse: Textual Analysis for Social Research*. London: Routledge.

Farquhar, Dion. 1996. *The Other Machine: Discourse and Reproductive Technologies*. London: Routledge.

Feasey, Rebecca. 2013. "From Soap Opera to Reality Programming: Examining Motherhood, Motherwork and the Maternal Role on Popular Television." *Imaginations: Journal of Cross-Cultural Image Studies* 4 (2): 25–46.

Feasey, Rebecca. 2015. *Mothers on Mothers: Maternal Readings of Popular Television*. Edinburgh: Edinburgh University Press.

Feuer, Jane. 1983. "The Concept of Live Television: Ontology as Ideology." In *Regarding Television*, edited by Ann Kaplan. Frederick, MD: University Publications of America.

Finding Nemo. 2003. Directed by Andrew Stanton, Lee Unkrich and written by Andrew Stanton, Bob Peterson, David Reynolds. Film. Los Angeles, CA: Walt Disney.

Finkelstein, Joanne. 1990. "Biomedicine and Technocratic Power." *Hastings Center Report* 20: 13–16. https://doi.org/10.2307/3562760.

Finley, Tara. 2015. "Organizer Says Black Residents Were 'Left To Die' After Hurricane Katrina." *Huffington Post US*, 25 August. http://www.huffington-post.com/entry/organizer-says-black-residents-were-left-to-die-after-hurri-cane-katrina_us_55dc805be4b04ae497046f9c.

Firestone, Shulamith. 1970. *Dialectic of Sex: The Case for a Feminist Revolution*. New York: Naomi Wolf.

Flavin, Jeanne, and Lynn Paltrow. 2010. "Punishing Pregnant Drug-Using Women: Defying Law, Medicine, and Common Sense." *Journal of Addicted Diseases* 29 (2): 231–244. https://doi.org/10.1080/10550881003684830.

Franklin, Sarah. 1990. "Deconstructing Desperateness': The Social Construction of Infertility in Popular Representations of New Reproductive Technologies" In *The New Reproductive Technologies*, edited by Maureen McNeil. London: Palgrave Macmillan.

Franklin, Sarah. 1991. "Fetal Fascinations: New Dimensions to the Medical-Scientific Construction of Fetal Personhood." In *Off-Centre: Feminism and Cultural Studies*, edited by Sarah Franklin, Celia Lury, and Jackie Stacey. Hammersmith: HarperCollins.

Franklin, Sarah, and Maureen McNeil. 1988. "Reproductive Futures: Recent Literature and Current Debates on Reproductive Technologies." *Feminist Studies* 14 (3): 545–561.

Friedman, May. 2014. "*Beyond MILF*: Exploring Sexuality and Feminism in Public Motherhood." *Atlantis* 36 (2): 49–60.
Frith, Simon. 1983. "Pleasures of the Hearth". *In Formations of Pleasure*. Paul Keegan. London: Routledge.
Gentile, Kate. 2011. "What About the Baby?' The New Cult of Domesticity and Media Images of Pregnancy." *Studies in Gender and Sexuality* 12 (1): 38–58.
Gerbner, George, Larry Gross, Michael Morgan, and Nancy Signorielli. 1986. *Living with Television*. Hillsdale, NJ: Lawrence Erlbaum Associates.
Gill, Rosalind. 2007. "Postfeminist Media Culture: Elements of Sensibility." *European Journal of Cultural Studies* 10 (2): 147–166.
Gill, Rosalind, and Elena Herdieckerhoff. 2006. "Rewriting the Romance: New Femininities in Chick Lit?" *Feminist Media Studies* 6 (4): 487–504.
Giuliana & Bill. 2009–2014. Executively produced by Alastair Surprise, Robert Sizemore. TV programme. Los Angeles, CA: E!.
Given, Lisa. 2008. *The Sage Encyclopedia of Qualitative Research Methods*. Los Angeles: Sage.
Goldenberg, Suzanne. 2017. "Rescued from Katrina, New Life for a Frozen Embryo." *The Guardian*, January 16. https://www.theguardian.com/world/2007/jan/16/hurricanekatrina.usa.
Gorton, Kristyn. 2009. *Media Audiences*. Edinburgh: Edinburgh University Press.
Grossberg, Larry. 1997. *Bringing It All Back Home: Essays on Cultural Studies*. Durham: Duke University Press.
Grosz, Elizabeth. 1994. *Volatile Bodies: Toward a Corporeal Feminism (Theories of Representation and Difference)*. Indiana: Indiana University Press.
Gupta, Jyotsna Agnihotri, and Annemiek Richters. 2008. "Embodied Subjects and Fragmented Objects: Women's Bodies, Assisted Reproduction Technologies and the Right to Self-Determination." *Journal of Bioethical Inquiry* 5 (4): 239–249.
Halberstam, Judith. 2011. *The Queer Art of Failure*. Durham: Duke University Press.
Halberstam, Judith. 2013. *Gaga Feminism: Sex, Gender and the End of Normal*. Boston: Beacon Press.
Hall, Stuart. 1973. *Encoding and Decoding in Television Discourse*. University of Birmingham: Centre for Contemporary Cultural Studies.
Hall, Stuart. 1997. *Representation: Cultural Representation and Signifying Practices*. London: Sage.
Hall, Radclyffe. 2014. *Well of Loneliness*. New ed. Ware: Wordsworth Editions.
Halperin, David. 2003. "The Normalization of Queer Theory." *Journal of Homosexuality* 45 (2–4): 339–343.
Han, Sallie. 2008. "Seeing Like a Family: Fetal Ultrasound Images and Imaginings of Kin." In *Imagining the Fetus the Unborn in Myth, Religion, and*

Culture, edited by Vanessa Sasson and Jane Marie Law. New York: Oxford University Press.

Haraway, Donna. 1988. "Situated Knowledges: The Science Question in Feminism and the Privilege of Partial Perspective." *Feminist Studies* 14 (3): 575. https://doi.org/10.2307/3178066.

Haraway, Donna. 2010. *Simians, Cyborgs, and Women*. New York, NY: Routledge.

Hartley, John. 1999. *Uses of Television*. London: Routledge.

Hewlett, Sylvia Anne. 2002. *Baby Hunger: The New Battle for Motherhood*. London: Atlantic.

Hill, Anette. 2004. *Realty TV Audience and Popular Factual Television*. London: Routledge.

Hirsch, Marianne. 1997. *Family Frames: Photography, Narrative, and Postmemory*. Cambridge: Harvard University Press.

Holland, Janet, and Caroline Ramazangolu. 2002. *Feminist Methodology: Challenges and Choices*. London: Sage.

Hollinger, Joan. 1984. "From Coitus to Commerce: Legal and Social Consequences of Noncoital Reproduction." *Reform* 18: 865–932.

Holmes, Su, and Deborah Jermyn. 2003. *Understanding Reality TV*. New York: Routledge.

Human Fertilisation & Embryology Authority. 2018. *Fertility Treatment 2014–2016*. https://www.hfea.gov.uk/media/2563/hfea-fertility-trends-and-figures-2017-v2.pdf. Accessed 2 January 2019.

Johnsen, Dawn E. 1986. "The Creation of Fetal Rights: Conflicts with Women's Constitutional Rights to Liberty, Privacy, and Equal Protection." Articles by Maurer Faculty. Paper 905.

Jones, Ellen E. 2017. "Empty Nests: Why Has TV Become Obsessed with Surrogate Mothers?" *The Guardian*, August 14. https://www.theguardian.com/tv-and-radio/2017/aug/14/top-of-the-lake-handmaids-tale-tv-obsessed-surrogate-mothers-infertility-parenting.

Kaplan, Anne. 1992. *Motherhood and Representation: The Mother in Popular Culture and Melodrama*. London: Routledge.

Kaplan, Anne. 1994. "Manifest Domesticity." *American Literature* 70 (3): 581–606, https://doi.org/10.2307/2902710.

Kavka, Misha. 2008. *Reality Television, Affect and Intimacy*. Hampshire: Palgrave Macmillan.

Kitzinger, Jenny. 1994. "The Methodology of Focus Groups: The Importance of Interaction Between Research Participants." *Sociology of Health & Illness* 16 (1): 103–121.

Kitzinger, Jenny. 2004. "The Methodology of Focus Groups: The Importance of Interaction Between Research Participants." *Sociology of Health and Illness* 16 (1): 103–121. https://doi.org/10.1111/1467-9566.ep11347023.

Lam, Carla. 2015. *New Reproductive Technologies and Disembodiment.* 1st ed. Abingdon: Routledge.
Lasch, Christopher. 1991. *The Culture of Narcissism.* New ed. New York: Norton.
Laverne & Shirley. 1976–1983. Created by Lowell Ganz, Garry Marshall, Mark Rothman. TV programme. Los Angeles, CA: Miller-Milkis.
Leibovitz, Annie. 1991. *Vanity Fair, More Demi Moore.*
Lester, Barry, Lynne Andreozzi, and Lindsey Appiah. 2004. "Substance Use During Pregnancy: Time for Policy to Catch Up with Research." *Harm Reduction Journal* 1 (1): 5.
Littler, Jo. 2013. "The Rise of the 'Yummy Mummy': Popular Conservatism and the Neoliberal Maternal in Contemporary British Culture." *Communication, Culture and Critique* 6 (2): 227–243. https://doi.org/10.1111/cccr.12010.
Longhurst, Rebecca. 2000. "Corporeographies of Pregnancy: Bikiki Babes." *Environment and Planning D: Society and Space* 18 (4): 453–472.
Losco, Joseph. 1989. "Fetal Abuse: An Exploration of Emerging Philosophical, Legal, and Social Policy Issues." *Political Research Quarterly* 42 (2): 265–286.
MacKinnon, Barbara. 2000. *Ethics: Theory and Contemporary Issues.* 3rd ed. Belmont, CA: Wadsworth Publishing.
Mad Men. 2007–2015. Created by Matthew Weiner. TV programme. Santa Monica, CA: Lionsgate.
Massumi, Brian. 2002. *Parables for the Virtual.* Durham, NC: Duke University Press.
Matthews, Sandra, and Laura Wexler. 2000. *Pregnant Pictures.* New York: Routledge.
McCarthy, Anna. 2001. *Ambient Television: Visual Culture and Public Space.* Durham, DC: Duke University Press.
McRobbie, Angela. 2004. "Post Feminism and Popular Culture." *Feminist Media Studies* 4 (3): 255–264.
Ministry of Justice Family Court. 2015. *Cafcass Study of Parental Order Applications Made in 2013/2014.* https://www.evidence.nhs.uk/document?id=1964928&returnUrl=Search%3Fpa%3D4%26q%3DCafcass%26s%3DDate&q=Cafcass. Accessed 4 July 2017.
Mittell, Jason. 2004. *Genre and Television: From Cop Shows to Cartoons in American Culture.* New York: Routledge.
Morley, David. 1980. *The Nationwide Audience.* London: British Film Institute.
Morley, David. 2006. "Unanswered Questions in Audience Research." *The Communication Review* 9 (2): 101–121.
Murdock, Anna. 1990. "Off the Treadmill—Leaving an IVF Programme Behind." In *The Baby Machine: Reproductive Technology and the Commercialisation of Motherhood,* edited by Jocelyn Scutt. London: Merlin Press.

Murray, Susan, and Laurie Ouellette. 2008. *Reality TV: Remaking Television Culture*. New York: New York University Press.

Naficy, Hamid. 1989. "Television Intertextuality and the Discourse of the Nuclear Family." *Journal of Film and Video* 41 (4): 42–59.

Nelson, Jennifer. 2003. *Women of Color and the Reproductive Rights Movement*. New York: New York University Press.

Nightingale, Virginia. 1996. *Studying Audiences: The Shock of the Real*. London: Routledge.

Oaks, Laurie. 2000. "Smoke-Filled Wombs and Fragile Fetuses: The Social Politics of Fetal Representation." *Signs* 26 (1): 63–108.

O'Donohoe, Stephanie. 2006. "Yummy Mummies: The Clamor of Glamour in Advertising to Mother." *Advertising & Society Review* 7 (3): 1–21.

Office for National Statistics. 2016. *Childbearing for Women Born in Different Years*. https://www.ons.gov.uk/peoplepopulationandcommunity/birthsdeathsandmarriages/conceptionandfertilityrates/bulletins/childbearingforwomenbornindifferentyearsenglandandwales/2015. Accessed 10 August 2017.

Oliver, Kelly. 1997. *Family Values: Subjects Between Nature and Culture*. New York: Routledge.

Oliver, Kelly. 2012. *Knock Me Up, Knock Me Down*. New York: Columbia University Press.

Pee-wee's Big Adventure. 1985. Directed by Tim Burton and written by Phil Hartman, Paul Reubens, Michael Varhol. Film. Burbank, CA: Warner Bros.

Petchesky, Rosalind. 1987. "The Power of Visual Culture and the Politics of Reproduction." *Feminist Studies* 13 (2): 263–292.

Petchesky, Rosalind. 1998. "Introduction". In *Negotiating Reproductive Rights: Women's Perspectives Across Countries and Cultures*, edited by Rosalind Petchesky and Karen Judd. New York: Palgrave Macmillan.

Pfeffer, Naomi, and Anne Woollett. 1983. *The Experience of Infertility*. London: Virago.

Plant, Sadie. 1996. "The Future Looms: Weaving Women and Cybernetics." In *Cyberspace/Cyberbodies/Cyberpunk: Cultures of Technological Embodiment*, edited by Mike Featherstone and Richard Burrows. London: Sage.

Press, Andrea. 1991. *Women Watching Television: Gender, Class, and Generation in the American Television Experience*. Philadelphia: University of Pennsylvania Press.

Pridmore-Brown, Michele. 2009. "Annie Lebovitz's Queer Consumption of Motherhood." *Women's Studies Quarterly* 37 (3–4): 81–95.

Private Life. 2018. Directed and written by Tamara Jenkins. Film. New York: Likely Story.

Radway, Janice. 1983. "Women Read the Romance: The Interaction of Text and Context." *Feminist Studies* 9 (1): 53–78.

Radway, Janice. 1992. *Reading the Romance: Women, Patriarchy, and Popular Literature*. 2nd ed. Chapel Hill, NC: University North Carolina.
Rand, Erin. 2014. *Reclaiming Queer: Activist and Academic Rhetorics of Resistance*. Alabama: University of Alabama Press.
Rich, Adrienne. 1980. "Compulsory Heterosexuality and Lesbian Existence." *Signs: Journal of Women in Culture and Society* 5 (4): 631–660.
Rich, Adrienne. 1996. *Of Woman Born: Motherhood as Experience and Institution*. Reissue. New York: W.W. Norton.
Roberts, Dorothy. 1996. "Race and the New Reproduction." *Faculty Scholarship at Penn Law*. 1154.
Roberts, Dorothy. 2000. *Killing the Black Body: Race, Reproduction, and the Meaning of Liberty*. New York: Vintage Books.
Roberts, Dorothy. 2014. "Complicating the Triangle of Race, Class and State: The Insights of Black Feminists." *Ethnic and Racial Studies* 37 (10): 1776–1782. https://doi.org/10.1080/01419870.2014.931988.
Robinson, James, and Thomas Skill. 2001. "Four Decades of Families on Television: A Demographic Profile, 1950–1989." In *Television and the American Family*, edited by Alison Bryant. 1st ed. New York: Routledge.
Rose, Hilary. 1994. *Love, Power and Knowledge: Towards a Feminist Transformation of the Sciences*. Cambridge: Polity Press.
Katz Rothman, Barbara. 2000. *Recreating Motherhood*. 2nd ed. New Jersey: Rutgers University Press.
Rowland, Robyn. 1992. *Living Laboratories: Women and Reproductive Technologies*. London: Lime Tree.
Rules of Engagement. 2007–2013. Created by Tom Hertz. TV programme. New York: CBS.
Sandelowski, Margarete. 1990. "Fault Lines: Infertility and Imperiled Sisterhood." *Feminist Studies* 16 (1): 33.
Sawicki, Janet. 1992. *Disciplining Foucault: Feminism, Power, and the Body*. New York: Routledge.
Schlichter, Annette. 2004. "Queer at Last? Straight Intellectuals and the Desire for Transgression." *GLQ: A Journal of Lesbian and Gay Studies* 10 (4): 543–564.
Scutt, Joceyln. 1990. *The Baby Machine: Reproductive Technology and the Commercialisation of Motherhood*. London: Merlin Press.
Seinfeld. 1989–1998. Created by Larry David and Jerry Seinfeld. TV programme. Los Angeles, CA: West-Shapiro.
Shira, Gabriel, Elaine Paravati, Melanie C. Green, and Jason Flomsbee. 2018. "From Apprentice to President: The Role of Parasocial Connection in the Election of Donald Trump." *Social Psychological and Personality Science* 9 (3): 299–307.
Silverstone, Roger. 1994. *Television and Everyday Life*. London: Routledge.

Skeggs, Beverley. 1997. *Formations of Class and Gender: Becoming Respectable.* London: Sage.

Skeggs, Beverley. 2005. "The Making of Class and Gender Through Visualizing Moral Subject Formation." *Sociology* 39 (5): 965–982.

Skeggs, Beverley. 2009. "The Moral Economy of Person Production: The Class Relations of Self-Performance on 'Reality' Television." *The Sociological Review* 57 (4): 626–644.

Skeggs, Beverley, and Helen Wood. 2011. *Reality Television and Class.* London: British Film Institute.

Skeggs, Beverley, and Helen Wood. 2012. *Reacting to Reality Television, Performance, Audience and Value.* Oxon: Routledge.

Skeggs, Beverley, Nancy Thumim, and Helen Wood. 2008. "'Oh Goodness, I am Watching Reality TV': How Methods Make Class in Audience Research." *European Journal of Cultural Studies* 11 (1): 5–24.

Slagle, Anthony. 1995. "In Defense of Queer Nation: From *Identity Politics* to a *Politics of Difference.*" *Western Journal of Communication* 59 (2): 85–102. https://doi.org/10.1080/10570319509374510.

Smith, Murray. 1995. *Engaging Characters: Fiction, Emotion and the Cinema.* Oxford: Clarendon Press.

Some Like It Hot. 1959. Directed by Billy Wilder and written by Billy Wilder, I.A.L. Diamond. Film. Los Angeles, CA: Ashton.

Spigel, Lynn. 2005. "TV's Next Season?" *Cinema Journal* 45 (1): 83–90.

Stanworth, Michelle. 1987. *Reproductive Technologies: Gender, Motherhood, Medicine.* Cambridge: Polity Press.

Statista. 2019. *Average Daily TV Viewing Time Per Person in Selected Countries Worldwide in 2016.* https://www.statista.com/statistics/276748/average-daily-tv-viewing-time-per-person-in-selected-countries/. Accessed 2 February 2019.

Taylor, Janelle. 1992. "The Public Fetus and the Family Car: From Abortion Politics to a Volvo Advertisement." *Public Culture* 4 (2): 67–80.

Taylor, Lisa, and Andrew Willis. 1999. *Media Studies: Texts, Institutions and Audiences.* Oxford: Blackwell.

Taylor, Lisa, and Helen Wood. 2008. "Feeling Sentimental About Television and Audiences." *Cinema Journal* 47 (3): 141–151, Project MUSE.

Teman, Tilly. 2005. *Birthing a Mother: The Surrogate Body and the Pregnant Self.* Berkeley: University of California Press.

The Handmaid's Tale. 2017–present. Created by Bruce Miller. Written by Margaret Atwood. TV programme. Channel 4.

The New Normal. 2012–2013. Created by Elodie Keene, Max Winkler, Ryan Murphy. TV programme. New York: NBC.

Thomas, Calvin. 2000. *Straight with a Twist: Queer Theory and the Subject of Heterosexuality.* Champaign: University of Illinois Press.

Thompson, Charis. 2005. *Making Parents: The Ontological Choreography of Reproductive Technologies*. Cambridge, MA: MIT Press.
Throsby, Karen. 2004. *When IVF Fails: Feminism, Infertility and the Negotiation of Normal*. Basingstoke: Palgrave.
Todorov, Tzvetan. 1990. *Genres in Discourse*. Cambridge: Cambridge University Press.
Top of the Lake: China Girl. 2017. Directed by Jane Campion and written by Jane Campion, Gerard Lee. TV programme. London: BBC2.
Treadwell, Mead. 1972. "Is Abortion Black Genocide?" *Family Planning Perspectives* 4 (1): 4–5.
Winddance Twine, France. 2011. *Outsourcing the Womb: Race, Class, and Gestational Surrogacy in a Global Market*. New York: Routledge.
Tyler, Imogen. 2001. "Skin-Tight: Celebrity, Pregnancy and Subjectivity." In *Thinking Through the Skin*, edited by Sara Ahmed, and Jackie Stacey. London: Routledge.
Tyler, Imogen. 2008. "Why the Maternal Now?" Published by the Department of Sociology, Lancaster University, Lancaster LA1 4YT, UK. http://www.lancs.ac.uk/fass/sociology/papers/tylerwhythematernalnow.pdf.
Tyler, Imogen. 2011. "Pregnant Beauty: Maternal Femininities Under Neoliberalism." In *New Femininities: Postfeminism, Neoliberalism and Subjectivity,* edited by Rosalind Gill and Christina Scharff. London: Palgrave Macmillan.
Uricchio, William. 2005. "Television's Next Generation: Technology/Interface Culture/Flow." In *Television After TV: Essays on a Medium in Transition,* edited by Lyn Spigel and Jan Olsson. Durham: Duke University Press, 2005.
Wacjman, Judy. 1991. *Feminism Confronts Technology*. Cambridge: Polity Press.
Walker, Janet. 1982. "Feminist Critical Practice: Female Discourse in Mildred Pierce." *Film Reader* 5: 164–172.
Warner, Michael. 1993. *Fear of a Queer Planet: Queer Politics and Social Theory*. Minneapolis: University of Minnesota Press.
Warner, Michael. 1999. *The Trouble with Normal*. Cambridge, MA: Harvard University Press.
Weir, Sara, and Constance Faulkner. 2004. *Voices of a New Generation*. Boston, MA: Pearson.
Wilkinson, Sue. 1999. "Focus Groups: A Feminist Method." *Psychology of Women Quarterly* 23 (2): 221–244.
Wilkinson, Sue. 2004. "Focus Group Research." In *Qualitative Research: Theory, Method, and Practice*, edited by David Silverman. Thousand Oaks, CA: Sage.
Williams, Linda. 1991. "Film Bodies: Gender, Genre, and Excess." *Film Quarterly* 44 (4): 2–13.
Winch, Alison. 2012. "We Can Have It All." *Feminist Media Studies* 12 (1): 69–82.

Wood, Helen. 2009. *Talking with Television: Women, Talk Shows, and Modern Self-Reflexivity.* Champaign: University of Illinois Press.

World Record Egg. 2019. "Let's Set a World Record Together and Get the Most Liked Post on Instagram. Beating the Current World Record Held by Kylie Jenner (18 million)! We Got This." Instagram. January 4. https://www.instagram.com/p/BsOGulcndj-/.

Yep, Gust. 2004. *Queer Theory and Communication: From Disciplining the Queers, to Queering the Disciplines(s)*. New York: Routledge.

Zajonc, Robert. 2000. "Feeling and Thinking: Closing the Debate Over the Independence of Affect." In *Feeling and Thinking: The Role of Affect in Social Cognition,* edited by Joseph Paul Forgas. Cambridge: Cambridge University Press.

CHAPTER 2

I Want a Baby! Baby Hunger and the Desire for a Genetic Child

This chapter examines the infertile intended mothers and their surrogates in *Giuliana & Bill* and *Coronation Street*. A variety of texts have been engaged with for this project, to explore how different genres articulate the practice of surrogacy through the genre's 'mode of address' (Feuer 1983, 17). This 'address' describes how audiences are engaged with through the sequencing of camera shots, dialogue, the positioning of actors within the scenes, and in some instances, audio use. This address structures the style of genre and emotion in the text—a key aim being to elicit responses from viewers. This will be explored in this chapter, and throughout the book.

Giuliana & Bill has been selected as a key text due to how the hunger for a genetic child steers the narrative. *Coronation Street* as a text is more complex, as the surrogacy storyline is one of multiple strands. *Giuliana & Bill* is a reality TV show about real people that follows the relationship and life of E! News host Giuliana and her husband Bill, winner of business game show, *The Apprentice*. A core storyline that emerges in Season 2 is that Giuliana has difficulty conceiving. After several miscarriages and failed IVF, she then discovers she has breast cancer, which halts any further treatment. She and Bill then engage a gestational surrogate to carry their genetic child. Their son Duke was born in Season 5.

Coronation Street is a fictional soap opera which follows character Tina when she becomes a surrogate for her neighbours, Izzy and Gary. Izzy is unable to conceive naturally due to her disability preventing her carrying

L. Le Vay, *Surrogacy and the Reproduction of Normative Family on TV*, Palgrave Studies in Science and Popular Culture,
https://doi.org/10.1007/978-3-030-17570-2_2

a foetus to term. Izzy's father engages Tina to be their surrogate, which helps her pay off a debt. After giving birth, Tina exercises her legal rights as the birth mother by reneging on the surrogacy agreement. She bonds with the child, Jake, and keeps him. After much emotional turmoil between the two parties, Tina eventually returns Jake to the intended parents, Izzy and Gary.

In these texts, the desire to acquire a genetic child materialises through what has been described as a baby hunger (Davitz 1984; Hewlett 2002; Kaplan 1992). It has been suggested that baby hunger has affected many professional, educated, predominantly white women, who have delayed childbearing due to a long period in higher education and/or getting established in a career (Bell 2010; Briggs 2017; Hewlett 2002; Sandelowski and de Lacy 2002). This resonates with Briggs' (2017) discussion of delayed childbearing, and how reproductive technologies like IVF have 'stepped into the breach, promising that this was a problem you could buy your way out of' (2017, 16). This notion of being able to buy one's fertility, and/or a baby, is explored further on. Economist Sylvia Anne Hewlett (2002) proposes that this baby hunger has an obsessive nature that can disrupt home and work life. Others, such as Susan Faludi (1993) argue that such anxieties are fuelled by the media, through an anti-feminist rhetoric. In all of the texts in focus, baby hunger steers the narrative, as all the female protagonists are infertile, and turn to reproductive technologies as a problem-solver.

Brooke Weihe Edge (2014) describes the infertility storyline in *Giuliana & Bill* as a 'backdoor reality' (2014, 875), when unexpected life occurrences guide the show's content. Edge argues that bringing infertility issues into mainstream viewing is positive, as it 'provides opportunities for informing audiences about infertility and its treatments, and potentially doing the same for other taboo topics' (2014, 873).

In contrast to Giuliana, Izzy in *Coronation Street* is working class. She sews underwear in a local factory. Izzy's desire for a child exhibits soap opera's central themes of motherhood and family (Brunsdon 1997; Gledhill 1987; Mumford 1991, 1995; Williams 1984). Her character, in relation to her struggles with infertility and miscarriages, demonstrates British soap opera's convention of social realism by making culturally visible social issues in the everyday lives of ordinary people (Couldry 2002; Dhoest 2005). This will be explored in more depth in relation to American TV media products further on. However, despite the differences, Izzy is also desperate for a genetic child. For this discussion, baby hunger will be examined through the lens of the disciplinary power of reproductive technologies (Farquhar 1996; Sawicki 1992). Michel Foucault (1977) proposed that disciplinary power materialises through the surveillance and monitoring of deviant bodies, such as those in a prison or mental institution. He believed this form of power is wielded as a rehabilitation tool, aimed to render the individual more productive, and more useful to society. Foucault claimed that only through this disciplinary process of normalisation could defective characteristics be ironed out.

Feminist Foucauldians Jana Sawicki (1992) and Dion Farquhar (1996) argue that reproductive technologies are a disciplinary practice, through the fixing of abnormalities to become a productive and useful subject—in this context, biological reproduction. However, Sawicki and Farquhar also propose that this form of power is not violent, or repressive, as they believe women are not *forced* to undergo treatment. They claim that reproductive technologies' power *incites* desire in active subjects, in their quest to become mothers. However, I argue that through popular cultural discourses this desire is mediated as accessible to a specific category of user, one who is white, heterosexual, married, professional and educated, predominantly in her later childbearing years (Franklin 1990; Hewlett 2002). This makes invisible, or renders deviant, other categories of users, which Farquhar describes as 'Other Mothers' (1996, 73)—single women, lesbians, women of colour, disabled women—and homosexuals. This concept of 'Other Mothers' will be applied at points throughout the book, primarily in the discussion of disabled intended mother Izzy in *Coronation Street* (this chapter), in the analysis of black adoptive mother Rocky in *The New Normal* (Chapter 3), and lesbian surrogate Brenda in *Rules of Engagement* (Chapter 4). It is important to highlight here that race theorist Patricia Hill Collins (2006) has also employed the term 'Othermother' (2006, 152) to describe women who share childcare in African American communities, a support system between women for survival. This will be explored in the discussion of fictive kinship in Chapter 5.

As highlighted in the previous chapter, Sarah Franklin (1990) identifies a discourse of desperateness in her study of the social construction of infertility in popular news representations, which in addition to Sawicki and Farquhar will aid these discussions. As Franklin proposes: 'Despite the fact that "desperateness" need not necessarily result from infertility, it is consistently the primary frame of reference within the popular representations of infertility' (1990, 204). Franklin also claims that this form of desperateness echoes those found in popular romance narratives, where in most stories the heroine seeks romance and protection by a man. The romance genre will be discussed further in Chapters 3 and 4. I argue that these discourses of desperateness in relation to narratives of infertility can be identified in *Giuliana & Bill* and *Coronation Street*, through the characters' desire to acquire a genetic child, through any means possible. Or, in Tina's case in *Coronation Street*, a yearning to keep the child she bonded with through surrogate pregnancy, despite no genetic relation. It is important to emphasise how important media narratives are to the fertility industry, as Farquhar explains:

> Contemporary medical narratives often depend on popular narratives for legitimation as well as for the dissemination of information about new technologies. Popular discourse adapts, reworks and constructs ARTs [assisted reproductive technologies] according to the uses and satisfactions it reports. These representations are often contradictory, sometimes challenging and other times reinforcing dominant conservative views of maternity, family, nature… (1996, 66)

I propose that the winner/loser binary can be identified in these shows' narratives—in this context the genetic mother (intended mother) being the winner, the surrogate being the loser. In addition, I also argue that Sara Ahmed's (2010) 'happy objects' and Lauren Berlant's (2011) 'cruel optimism' are concepts that will aid the analysis.

For Ahmed, happy objects are objects that good feelings are directed towards, and to follow their direction will lead us to happiness. These objects are end-orientated and can be pleasurable by evoking feelings of happiness before the object has been encountered. Happy objects, aside from the genetic baby in this discussion, can also be the vision of the happy family, the family home and all the objects that reside within it—such as the display of family photographs. However, Ahmed also highlights that these happy objects can also be obstacles to one's happiness, as they preserve the fantasy of what one needs to be happy, and which therefore become unhappy objects.

Berlant's cruel optimism in relation to objects is similar, in the sense that the objects of desire can be both enabling and disabling. For Berlant, optimism can be found in the attachments to not just objects, but to people, places, norms and practices, which promise, 'a change that's gonna come' (2011, 2). Where Ahmed's happy objects are end-orientated, and symbolic of future stepping-stones into the happy horizon, Berlant's objects of desire are based in the present, as a 'process of emergence' (2011, 7). Berlant believes these objects are cruelly optimistic as they can be obstacles to one flourishing—problematic, risky, toxic. Yet, one remains attached to them. Berlant argues that one can only discover life's contentment when one can let go of the attachment. However, it is the attachments that hold one's optimism for the future, which is when it becomes cruel.

These tensions and attachments to objects of desire are central to these discussions, the objects of desire in this context being the genetic child and the creation of normative family. I argue that these representations reinforce the ideal of the normative nuclear family, which infer that families are only viewed as complete, and normalised, with the addition of children (Benkov 1994; Lehr 1999; Nelson 2007, 2009). These normative ideals also perpetuate the notion that a woman only become whole, and socially accepted, when she becomes a mother. Adrienne Rich (1980) claims this ideological process into motherhood takes place within a wider framework she calls a compulsory heterosexuality—socially and culturally constructed norms which she argues socialises women into heterosexual romance and marriage, distorting other possible options, such as lesbianism, in the process. Although this will be touched upon here, this will be explored further in Chapter 4.

In addition, what has emerged as poignant by the focus group participants is how the identities of the genetic mother (the intended mother) and the birth mother (the surrogate) are articulated differently, in relation to differing genre mechanisms, and how these mechanisms influence their understanding of the surrogacy practice through the evocation of empathy for key characters. Kristyn Gorton (2009) highlights the importance of such mechanisms in the ability to connect emotionally with audiences, not in terms of identification with the characters based purely on their shape, but through their engagement with the text. As Gorton emphasises: 'It is not simply that a viewer sees a character and *identifies* with them, rather it is a more complex process in which the emotional situation the character is in elicits a response while, at the same time, technical devices such as a close-up shot or music aids and develops this connection' (2009, 151). I argue that emotions connect—or as I explore in some cases do not connect, depending on the genre—with the female viewers through an affective register, which is created through how emotions are structured in the genre (Carroll 1990, 1996; Gorton

2009; Williams 1991). Furthermore, what has emerged as significant is how these representations also impact on how the participants view their own position as women, as mothers, non-mothers and pre-mothers.

Core themes that have emerged through the analysis of the focus group data are the value of motherhood and family in modern mainstream culture, the impact of choice that reproductive technologies have placed on a female subject diagnosed with infertility, and the sense of entitlement that is attached to certain bodies in this desire to reproduce—some which are visible, and some which are not. What has also materialised as significant is how the audiences were able to identify power imbalances between the intended mothers and their surrogates through not just the construction of the characters within the storylines, but through how they have been positioned on the screen. This, as I argue, drawing on Margarete Sandelowski (1990), creates voids between women through how infertility and motherhood have been shaped through culture.

To explore this desire for a genetic child that drives the narratives in both *Coronation Street* and *Giuliana & Bill*, a breadth of feminist work on emotions and affect, media representation, compulsory heterosexuality, infertility, reproductive technologies and race will be drawn on.

This chapter is divided into three parts. *Baby hunger* aims to examine the discourse of desperateness and ideologies of fulfilment in relation to the acquisition of a genetic child and the formation of normative family. *The winner gets it all* explores the impact of reproductive technologies on the female body in the context of disciplinary power and the winner/loser binary, and *Out of the frame* further illustrates this hierarchical division by identifying how privilege, status and power are attached to, and block, certain bodies, through narrative devices and genre techniques.

Baby Hunger

> I think that even still in this day and age a lot of women think that's what they need to do. Is that the best answer for them? I don't know.
>
> (Jackie, mixed mothers focus group, 2015)

Nancy Chodorow (1999) argued that women wanted children to not only add richness to their heterosexual relationships with men, which she believed some women viewed as lacking intensity and meaning, but to recreate their own relationships with their mothers. In response to this,

Rich (1980) proposed that Chodorow neglected an important factor in her theory. Rich argued that having children wasn't simply a strategy to fill an empty void, but was the result of dominant social forces, which she called compulsory heterosexuality—a force that directs women into heterosexual couplings, marriage and motherhood. This, she argued, could be identified throughout all aspects of society and culture, particularly in the ideology of heterosexual romance embedded in the images and narratives presented in fairy tales, film, TV, advertising and literature. Rich believed this was a form of cultural propaganda that wielded power over women, who were assumed heterosexual. Rich claimed that through this institution of heterosexuality, lesbian existence was blocked, and that to be heterosexual assured men's power over women—physically, emotionally and economically. This blocking of the lesbian existence will be discussed in Chapter 3, where I argue that natural pregnancy is represented as the normative ideal, over the non-normative surrogate pregnancy *and* the abnormality of infertility. In the analysis of *Baby Mama* and *Rules of Engagement* I argue that heterosexual love and the couple dyad enables natural pregnancy, against all odds—a miracle *pregnancy* (natural) rather than the miracle *baby* (technology), which is central to this discussion.

The idealisation of motherhood and the baby as an object of desire (the miracle) is the focus here. I argue that this drive towards motherhood, and the desire for and attainment of a genetic child, is also, as Rich (1980) described about heterosexuality, an assumptive norm that is central to a woman's identity, and that motherhood should be studied as a political institution, like heterosexuality. As Jackie (mixed mothers focus group) explained: 'I think that even still in this day and age a lot of women think that's what they need to do'. This indicates not just compulsory heterosexuality, but what I call a *compulsory motherhood*—the desire for motherhood, like heterosexuality, being the result of a control of consciousness, through cultural propaganda.

Giuliana's quest to become a mother has steered the narrative in *Giuliana & Bill* since the show launched in 2009. Echoing Hewlett's description of baby hunger, which she proposes is the result of delaying reproduction due to women's pursuit of a career, Giuliana took sole responsibility for her infertility. In an interview with *Health* magazine (Spencer 2012), Giuliana put her infertility down to, 'chasing a career instead of chasing guys' which echoes Hewlett's belief that the more successful the woman, the less likely she is to have a partner and baby. The cameras follow Giuliana and Bill to all the doctors' appointments, offering the audience intimate insights into the ordeals the couple face on the path to obtaining a genetic child. Giuliana has several miscarriages and becomes unwell with breast cancer. During the flashback sequence in 'Meet the Duke!' (Season 5, Episode 18), a collection of past clips is shown, illustrating the emotional roller coaster of their fertility journey. In one scene Giuliana is shown disintegrating into tears during a therapy session: 'I just feel like… why are we being punished in a way?' The responsibility of infertility frequently resides with the woman, often resulting in feelings of failure, punished for being defective and unfit for motherhood (Braverman 1997; Edge 2014; Throsby 2004). The disciplinary practice of reproductive technologies, which sets out to rectify these failings, will be explored in the following section.

This intimate filming style is core to the aesthetic style of reality TV, which also incorporates monologue-style interviews direct to camera. These methods attempt to provide an authentic frame by enabling viewers to have closer access to the character (Aslama and Pantti 2006). These monologues are interspersed with the observational documentary style of cinema verité—naturalistic, intimately filmed sequences, often on a hand-held camera (Nichols 1983, 1991). In these flashback scenes, Giuliana is shown sobbing to news of miscarriages or cancer to then being overjoyed at pregnancy news, which is followed, once again, by loss. In the later episodes, leading up to the birth of her genetic son, Giuliana is shown as over-animated, ecstatic.

It has been argued that displays of emotion create an illusion of intimacy, through this blurring of the public with the private, which allows the audience to feel close to their raw, naked feelings (Aslama and Pantti 2006; Schickel 2000). However, this 'being yourself' requires a performance as a 'half actor' which always presumes an audience—not acting up for the cameras, but 'acting out' (Kavka 2008, 97). This construction of intimacy also draws on the documentary's observational mode by showing 'the emotional experiences of individuals' (Nash 2011, 229).

The genre conventions of reality TV, much like soap opera, imply a female viewer, as the ideological framework encompasses romance, marriage and family life (Brunsdon 2000; Hobson 1982). Skeggs and Wood (2012) have argued, extending Jane Feuer's (1983) work on ideology and television, that 'it is not just in the mode of address that ideology operates, but in what that address asks the viewer *to do*' (2012, 228). In the context of the *Giuliana & Bill* footage shown in the viewing sessions, it can be proposed that the address was inviting the viewer to feel through 'emotion markers' (Smith 1999, 18)—textual cues specifically created to prompt an emotional response. This can be identified in Carla's (mixed mothers focus group) response to the text:

> Obviously, there are some moments of real, authentic emotion throughout that show, you know... filming someone finding out they're having a miscarriage is raw. So actually, that is going to, even if you are cynical and scathing, resonate on some level as it's a real thing, it's not acting, and that's why these kind of shows people engage with, as you're waiting for the real emotional crisis because that's the bit that makes it worth watching... You want to see people in pain or in great joy.
>
> (Carla, mixed mothers focus group, 2015)

Despite revealing a critical dislike for the show, the emotion markers embedded in the narrative prompted Carla to empathise with Giuliana's display of emotion, which Carla believed to a 'real thing'. This was crafted through the manipulation of affect that the mode of address asked her to 'do'—in this example, asked her to *feel.* As Gorton (2009) argues, in relation to how one's critical judgment of the reality TV genre can conflict with the emotional response: 'Many viewers find themselves crying during lifestyle or reality television despite their critical opinions of the programme... although viewers can be critical of these texts they also find themselves emotionally moved by them' (2009, 110). Alongside demonstrating this tension through her response, Carla was also able to describe the pleasure of engaging with displays of emotion on screen, particularly through reality TV's method of observing people in difficult emotional situations (Hill 2004).

While sympathising with Giuliana's miscarriage trauma, Carla was also describing the mechanism of the 'money shot'—a term appropriated from pornography by Laura Grindstaff (2002) which she applied to the baring all of emotions on talk show TV. Grindstaff uses this term to describe the moments when the show's participants express their emotions in visible terms 'for the pleasure, fascination, or repulsion of viewers... Like the orgasmic cum shot of pornographic films, the money shot of talk shows makes visible the letting go, of losing control' (2002, 20). This emotional release frequently emerges in *Giuliana & Bill*, which I propose is an expression of the desperateness of baby hunger. As family and marriage researcher Lois Davitz (1984) explains: 'The drive to have a baby unleashes a whole range of obsessive emotions a woman may never have had to face. When a woman has baby hunger, nothing else is as important to her as this inner drive to bear a child' (in Franklin 1990, 207).

Drawing on Berlant (2008, 2011) I propose that Giuliana's emotional displays not only reflect the desperateness that drives her baby hunger, but also highlight a discourse of disappointment, through her quest to become a mother. The attachment to the object of desire—the genetic child—being cruelly optimistic as it becomes a source of anxiety by being risky and problematic. In addition, Berlant also states that through this anxiety there is disappointment, which shares the binary with fulfilment, which work together and not as opposites. This is shown in Giuliana's proximity to the happy object (pregnancy, fulfilment), which is followed by loss (miscarriage, disappointment).

Berlant talks of the discourse of disappointment in relation to what she calls 'the female complaint' (2008, 13), which she argues drives women's desire to live for normative ideologies of love. This, she proposes, is transmitted through the sentimentally of the romance narrative, which is core to the construction of popular women's texts. Berlant claims that this desire for fulfilment is to be 'a *somebody* in the world, where the default is being a nobody' which can only be achieved through heterosexual love and the formation of family (2008, 3). This correlates with the notion that a woman is not complete until she becomes a mother, a theory that is rooted in the Cartesian nature/culture binary that associates women's bodies with nature, and therefore natural reproduction, an ideology of motherhood that has been entrenched in Western culture as core to woman's natural identity (Charlebois 2011; Lam 2015). This is explored in more depth in Chapter 4, alongside the proposition that the search for romantic love is being eclipsed by the search for a baby, the *future foetus* being a happy object embedded with affective value before its arrival. This I argue further illustrates the shift from compulsory *heterosexuality* to compulsory *motherhood*, the possession of the genetic child—and the arrival of the *future foetus*—symbolising a perfect end (Ahmed 2010).

The tales of desperateness, which lead to fulfilment, that Franklin identified in popular news stories also reflect Ahmed's notion of happy objects and the happy horizon, while following Tzvetan Todorov's (1990) narrative structure which advances from goal to the final equilibrium, which can be seen in *Giuliana & Bill*. The narrative unfolds like this: the goal (get the baby), equilibrium (turning to IVF to help create a family), disruption (miscarriages, breast cancer), resolution (engaging a surrogate to carry their genetic child), final equilibrium (birth of a baby boy, creating a family, becoming a mother). Similar narrative structures re-emerge in the analysis of *Baby Mama*, which is discussed in Chapter 4. As Franklin (1990) explains: 'The plot is structured around the tension between the desperate desire for a child and the biological inability to produce one. It is both an adventure story and a romance, in which a successful fight "against the odds" may end in "a dream come true"' (1990, 203). Although Franklin's analysis is drawn from news stories, the plot in *Giuliana & Bill* mirrors her findings.[1] It is important to highlight that despite the genre being named 'reality' TV, the articulation of Giuliana's experiences is still *mediated* and *constructed*—its authenticity in relation to soap opera discussed further on.

During the surrogate's labour in a Denver medical centre, Bill's mother and sister are pictured in a sequence of scenes, preparing a hotel suite for Giuliana and Bill's return to Chicago with their newborn son. These scenes provoked an interesting discussion between Laura and Rachel (non-mothers focus group):

> Rachel: I thought it was like, um, very much like… they kept showing the Four Seasons hotel… it felt like it was all about surface. A baby was actually, I thought, just a product. It felt it was something to enhance their life, like their life wasn't complete without a baby. And when they took the picture out, it was all surface, all staging – everything was acquired.
>
> Laura: A friend of mine went through 2-3 years of IVF and it crippled them financially, she was just like, "I want a baby", and it was weird. When we first met she never wanted kids, never wanted anything like that, then suddenly she was like (gasp sound) "I want a baby!" People tell you about that, suddenly your biological clock will kick in. I'm like "whatevs", but it actually happened to her.
>
> Rachel: There are probably millions of women like your friend that I would not attribute any of these criticisms to.
>
> Laura: I know! I know!
>
> Rachel: I'm not saying that, that she didn't *want* a baby; I'm just saying that it's being presented on a reality show.
>
> Laura: Of course! I was just saying we don't actually *know* how Giuliana feels.
>
> Rachel: I think that's a really good point, as I think… in all the American shows it's always *always* about the parents, and never about the baby, it's always me, me me… "I want a baby!" and "I can't have a baby!" What I got as a theme was that surrogacy is just a vehicle to get "what I want".
>
> (Rachel and Laura, non-mothers focus group, 2015)

Rachel stresses the notion that a family is not complete 'without a baby', which, as has been discussed, emphasises the inclusion of a genetic child to create the picture of the proper family (Barrett and McIntosh 1991). This echoes early twentieth-century beliefs that pairings that were unable to reproduce were seen as unfit and unnecessary, divorces granted out of court. In addition, Laura was able to make sense of Giuliana's experiences of infertility, although mediated, by relating the representation of baby hunger to a friend's experience, as well as her own, while recognising the codes and conventions of the reality TV genre. Kristina Engwall and Helen Peterson's (2013) observation about the silent body is identifiable in Laura's description of her friend's baby hunger, in relation to her own feelings of *not* desiring a child. They argue this is when the female subject has no desire to be a mother yet is still open to the possibility that a dormant maternal desire might wake up. As Laura stated: '... suddenly she was like (gasp sound) "I want a baby!"... Suddenly your biological clock will kick in'.

In contrast, Rachel was more concerned with how the surrogacy process was shaped within the show's narrative. She thought the way in which the gifts delivered to the hotel suite were shown off to the camera was distasteful. She argued that this made the production of a child through surrogacy appear like it was simply an object to be 'acquired'—a lifestyle commodity to be obtained. This resonates with Roberts (1995) argument that images of fertility treatment in the popular media are as constructed as white, 'the blue-eyed, blond-haired baby held up to television cameras as the precious product of a surrogacy arrangement' (1995, 210). The media construction of such images is discussed in more detail further on. Furthermore, this also reflects what Lisa Baraitser and Imogen Tyler (2010) have named a maternal market, a multi-billion-dollar industry, which not only trades in baby clothes and products, but also, 'fertility treatments, eggs, foetuses and children' (2010, 118). Furthermore, Rachel's observation of the baby as object in the context of consumer culture and the desire for a *specific* type of motherhood also evokes the figure of the yummy mummy—and her American sister, the MILF—in the shaping of Giuliana's character. As both Jo Littler (2013) and Stephanie O'Donohoe (2006) have argued, the yummy mummy is an aspirational maternal brand with economic currency, steered by white and class privilege. As Littler argues in relation to increasing birth rates in America: 'where there have been no improvements in welfare entitlements, the rise in births is usually simply put down to the wealthy having more babies' (2013, 8).

In her discussion Littler highlights the work of Haya El Nassa and Paul Overberg (2007) who suggest that in modern times, kids have become luxury goods. This is precisely what Rachel found the disturbing aspect of wealthy celebrities being able to buy a baby like a 'product'. I propose this, in the context of what has been described as a maternal market, indicates how reproductive technologies in America interconnect with contemporary capitalism, due to the political revolution of neoliberalism that emerged in the late seventies 'in which corporate America and Wall Street have reset government priorities to shrink spending on the well-being of actual humans' (Briggs 2017, 8–9). This link between austerity and reproductive assistance is explained in more detail below.

Laura Briggs claims that in America reproductive labour (birthing and caring for children/dependents, looking after the home) are irrefutably political. This she argues is because: 'When we are talking about the economy, we are talking about reproductive politics, because families and households are where we live our economic situation' (2017, 4). Continuing Karl Marx's work on changing family structures in relation to the birth of capitalism, Frederick Engels (2001) claimed that the family was as an active unit in constant evolution, developing to a higher stage of social form in relation to shifts in economic and political structures, such as the birth of industry, the growth and impact of private property and the materialisation and intervention of the state. Engels' aim through his analysis was to illuminate women's subordination within the monogamous coupling of the patriarchal family, which he claimed was founded to assure paternal lineage and the transfer of property. This he believed was a defining moment that was to shape family hierarchy. Although here is not the space to explore this work in detail, what is useful to recognise is how modern reproductive politics echoes his belief that the introduction of private property has created conditions to oppress women. Therefore, as I argue throughout this book, this underscores how nineteenth-century notions of domesticity and motherhood continue to re-emerge in contemporary culture, capitalism and state regulation.

Within political frameworks Briggs identifies a number of significant issues in relation to the development of family ideology, primarily through addressing 'the ferocious rise in business's power to define how we live' (2017, 120). Firstly, Briggs maintains that since the 1980s, the withdrawal of government support for the family in America and declining wages has been—and still is—fuelled by the politics of racial division, from Reagan to Trump, largely activated through the 'race-based shaming of supposedly irresponsible reproductive behavior' (2017, 189). As has been discussed, this is a rhetoric that has been shaped through the image of the idle and sexually promiscuous black welfare queen of the Reagan era. Continuing divisive politics, the current Trump administration champions white supremacy while promising financial stability through a nationalist agenda.

Secondly, through this new denationalised responsibility to support the family and low wages, women began to suffer from what she calls a 'structural infertility' (2017, 16). Briggs argues this type of infertility is the effect of women remaining in education and the workplace for longer, resulting in the fertility window slamming shut. This she proposes is due to the threat of economic insecurity *and* family unfriendly work environments, which has delayed reproduction.

However, as a result of this fragility more mothers are going back to work than ever before, which as it has been argued frames them as bad mothers—failures as women. This is due to women stepping outside of the domestic role and being away from their children (Borisoff 2005; Feasey 2017; Tincknell 2005). The perfect mother figure is becoming increasingly unattainable, which Rebecca Feasey (2015) argues enforces an ideology of motherhood which is 'intensive', demanding that women must devote all their time and be responsible for every aspect of their child's needs, while also finding it rewarding.

Where a door is shut and desperate individuals are trying to wedge it open to find happiness—in this case, happiness wrapped up in the form of a baby—commercial industries will step in with a solution, as long as it's profitable. Briggs claims that delayed reproduction has led to the upsurge in demand for assisted conception, fuelling a billion-dollar industry, the high cost of which not only deterring certain types of potential users (non-white, non-abled, non-married etc.) but feeding into a 'thriving neo-liberal debt market happy to exploit people's urgent desire for children' (2017, 110).

Briggs proposes this 'desire' has resulted in the emergence of fertility financing; bank loans aimed at the less wealthy—much like the over-zealous selling of sub-prime mortgages which contributed to America's economic crash of 2007. This finance offers those struggling with infertility the possibility of acquiring a child—like buying a car—despite the low success rates. This therefore results in more debt on top of the debt already accumulated through attaining an education and a home. Briggs is able to highlight that reproductive politics in America is intrinsically linked with the force of the right-wing movement which develops policies to reduce government support programmes for predominantly non-white poor people as a block to class progression, and a private/public benefits system 'haunted by eugenics' (2017, 107) which determines who has the right to have or not have children. As she identifies: 'Insurers pay for the poor to get birth control and for the rich to get IVF' (2017, 108).[2] The white *future foetus* must be saved. Contemporary capitalism to the rescue! This is especially poignant in the context of the Trump administration's antiquated position on women's reproductive rights, which impacts on both women *and* men's fundamental human rights to decide whether or not to have children; and which, drawing on Joanne Finkelstein (1990) I propose is a strategy by which to restore women to their normative biological destiny as mothers.

Giuliani in *Giuliani & Bill* (and the majority of the other childless characters analysed in this study) is representative of the delayed reproduction that Brigg's emphasises, alongside exhibiting the white privilege which Briggs claims enables access to assisted reproduction—and which fuels its growing demand—through the hunger for a child. In relation to this desire for a child, Rachel and Laura, in their earlier exchange, identified discourses of desperateness and disappointment in the narrative structure, through statements: 'I want a baby' (desperateness, the goal) and 'I can't have a baby' (disappointment, disruption). Furthermore, a discourse of emotional self-interest can be identified through Rachel recognising that surrogacy is being portrayed as a practice to get, 'what I want'—a 'luxury good' to be purchased (El Nasser and Overberg 2007). This describes the subject's feelings of pleasure before the *future foetus's* arrival, value *attached* to the happy object (Ahmed 2010) rather than having its own value in isolation. As Rachel commented: 'it's never about the baby, it's always me, me, me'.

The desire for fulfilment, which Berlant argues can be found in the safe and comfortable folds of normative family life, can be developed further here through Rachel's observation of how the picture of Bill as a child with his now deceased father was unwrapped and positioned by his mother and sister during the hotel suite scenes. The framed photograph (Fig. 2.1) was placed on a table facing the front door, accompanied by a toy—a symbolic welcome to the new parents when they arrive with their newborn son. This picture is positioned in a close-up shot for heightened emotional impact, which also performs as an 'emotion marker' (Smith

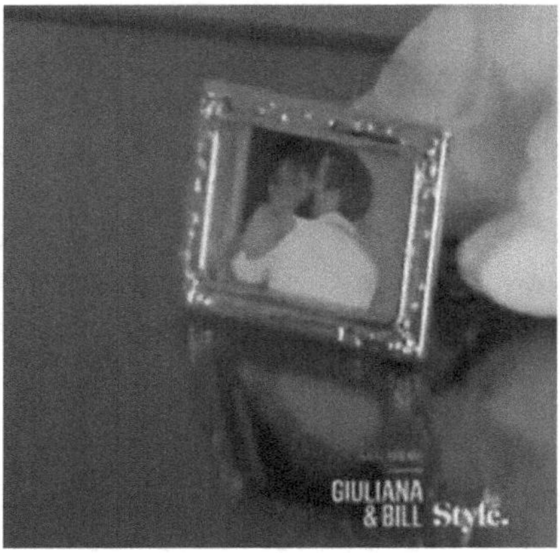

Fig. 2.1 *Giuliana & Bill*, Season 5, Episode 18, "Meet the Duke," Produced by Robert Sizemore, aired November 20, 2012 on E!, accessed July 21, 2017, E! 2009–2014, https://www.amazon.co.uk/gp/video/detail/B018YGPFEW?ref_=aiv_dp_season_select

1999, 18) to evoke a sentimental response. Although cognitive theory has traditionally been applied to film, Gorton (2009) argues it is also useful for television analysis. Such emotional mechanisms are constructed in the narrative to invite viewers to feel—they can either accept or reject such invites (Smith 2008).

However, for Rachel, this device didn't work. She felt these scenes were an act of 'staging' and 'surface', which resonated with Carla (mixed mothers focus group) who felt that viewing the show was like 'eating a bag of sweets, you know, you'll watch it and then go "urgh!"' As outlined by Noel Carroll (2008), the audience can only be led by the filmmaker to drink the water 'but the circuit is not completed until the audience drinks' (in Gorton 2009, 79). Gorton claims this doesn't always happen, which is demonstrated here.

In a later scene where the couple is at the hospital awaiting the arrival of their child, Giuliana, who is holding the camera, interviews an excited Bill. This further illustrates the influence of observational documentary's cinema verité, where the filmmaker's voice can often be heard to create a more situated presence (Nichols 1991). These scenes will be explored in more depth in the final section. Bill shares his excitement about the imminent arrival of his son by producing a picture of his father from his pocket (Fig. 2.2).

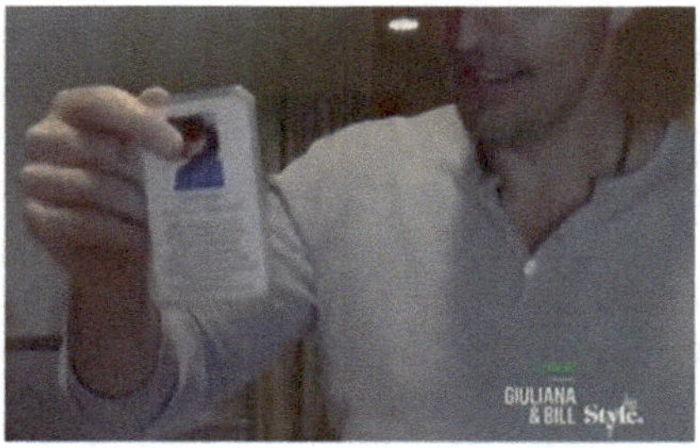

Fig. 2.2 *Giuliana & Bill*, Season 5, Episode 18, "Meet the Duke," Produced by Robert Sizemore, aired November 20, 2012 on E!, accessed July 21, 2017, E! 2009–2014, https://www.amazon.co.uk/gp/video/detail/B018YGPFEW?ref_=aiv_dp_season_select

He holds it up to the camera and says: 'I've got my good luck picture of my dad that I take to all important events' (Season 5, Episode 18: 'Meet the Duke!'). I propose that by displaying the photograph of his father held close to his body within this frame, this scene is signalling a family togetherness through evoking memory, bringing back into focus deceased family members. In her ethnographic work with women and family photographs, but which can be applied here, Gillian Rose (2010) argues that this togetherness through the display of a family photograph creates a domestic scene which keeps the family unit intact. Drawing on Ahmed (2006, 2010) and Marianne Hirsch (1997) I also suggest that this also chimes with the notion that photographs are rooted in modern family ideology which exhibit the value of genetic family cohesion through kinship objects, which includes, alongside photographs, objects such as the kitchen table that families gather around (Ahmed 2006). The visibility of these objects, therefore, producing the family as a happy object. Furthermore, this scene also suggests that photographs, more than the foetal image that has widely penetrated popular culture, has more cultural power over scientific visualisations (Taylor 1992), which 'can resurrect the dead or preserve lost love' (Petchesky 1987, 269).

Furthermore, the images of the father, and of father and son, are also symbolic of patrilineage, a genetic tie through male descent that is core to patriarchy. Barbara Katz Rothman (2000) argues that the development of reproductive technologies is based on 'the patriarchal focus on the male seed' (2000, 23). However, interestingly, the young women in the pre-mothers focus group didn't share Rachel's interpretation of these scenes as being inauthentic. They *did* accept the invitation to feel—they drank it in. During the viewing session, most of the women responded with comments such as, 'aw...' and 'how sweet!' This might be because they are younger, dependent on their families and still located within the family home, which could potentially heighten emotional bonds. I suggest that these younger women are yet to experience both emotional and geographical distance from the security of the family home (and their parents) as well as not being able to draw upon the range of experiences available to the older participants.

These photographs represent not just a hunger for the *future foetus* to arrive as a genetic child but displays the promise of happiness that is attached to the arrival of a very *specific* child—one that is white and male. In opposition to what Ahmed might argue, the kinship object of these photographs, in this context, *don't* do the work of keeping families together, as the family is not yet formed, but they *do* do the work to make families *happen*, as they point *towards* the happiness of the future family that is just over the horizon.

The Winner Gets It All

> The boundaries keep getting pushed, women aren't allowed, or can't say, actually, it's not going to happen, because they keep changing, the... you know... you can try that, try that, or try that.
>
> (Carla, mixed mothers focus group, 2015)

As outlined, Franklin proposes that stories of infertility are structured with winners and losers, which infer that there are 'happy endings for some and hopelessness for others' (1990, 204). Extending this, I argue that the characters affected by infertility in both shows are initially positioned as losers but are able to transform into winners through the intervention of the disciplinary practice of reproductive technologies, which enables the characters to achieve their biological destiny as women. As Farquhar (1996) explains: 'If a primary gender norm for women is "mother," then the extent to which reproductive technologies help reproductively impaired women achieve this identity is the extent to which they contribute to keeping women properly aligned in their gender role' (1996, 107). I also show the volatility of the winner/loser positions in these shows through how the narratives unfold, the tensions between the characters, and how the characters reposition.

Despite characters Izzy in *Coronation Street* and Giuliana in *Giuliana & Bill* being situated in different genres, produced in different countries, and portrayed as being from different backgrounds, the goal in the narratives are the same—to get a baby, through any means possible. The characters are driven by the desperateness of baby hunger, the winner/loser binary shaping both narratives. However, I propose this binary is more prominent in *Coronation Street* due to Tina being a popular character on the show before the appearance of the surrogacy storyline. Delphine, the gestational surrogate in *Giuliana & Bill*, appears later in the series, with minimal inclusion in the scenes. This has been read as exclusionary by the focus groups, which will be debated at the end of this chapter.

In this discussion, the transformative practice is surrogacy, which makes genetic motherhood possible for Izzy and Giuliana, despite the polarisation of their class. Izzy's character in *Coronation Street* is ordinary and working class—her father is a builder and she works in a factory. In addition to her infertility, Izzy is also an 'Other Mother' through disability. This contradicts arguments by a range of feminists who argue that reproductive technologies are only shown as accessible to the privileged white middle classes through the picture of the white mother cradling her miracle baby (Ceballo 1999; Farquhar 1996; Franklin 1990; Roberts 1995, 1996, 2000; Throsby 2004). However, what these representations *do* reflect is the exclusion of black women's bodies from having access, and being in proximity, to these technologies, which will be discussed further on.[3]

In both *Coronation Street* and *Giuliana & Bill* surrogacy is pursued as a last resort, after IVF fails—or in Izzy's case, when she decides not to attempt natural pregnancy after a miscarriage threatens her health. This evidences how the allure of reproductive technologies maintains the baby as a future goal. Drawing on Berlant (2008) this can be read as cruelly optimistic as it represents a 'cluster of promises' (2008, 23) that offers the prospect of a 'change that's gonna come' (2008, 1). As Carla pointed out: 'The boundaries keep getting pushed… you can try that, try that, or try that… '. This reflects Franklin's (1990) belief that due to the growth of reproductive choices, our choices also expand. Or as Carla stated: 'the carrot is constantly being dangled'. Sonja, Carrie and Nadra (mixed mothers focus group) had a revealing discussion about the desire for motherhood in relation to reproductive technologies:

Sonja: I think there's a theme through it all, of the society we live in, that by hook or by crook you will have it all, and the judgments which come with that. In previous times, you'd just be childless. This is all new ground, isn't it? Like what you, Lulu, were saying, that there's now a genre of movie called "mom-com". You know, so this whole issue of women waiting until they're older and infertility problems and things like that, and all the different ways there are these days to try and have a baby, it's coming with a whole new set of judgments and, erm, yeah…

Carrie: It creates so much unhappiness actually, because it says you're not really trying, and you're not valid if you don't have a child.

Nadra: I think that's really bad, yeah.

Carrie: That's what's interesting for me… 20 years ago it was like, oh, you can't have kids? That's such a shame, but there are a lot of other things you can do.

Nadra: You can crack on.

Carrie: Yeah, whereas now it's… you can do this, do this, or this – as that *must* be what you do. Women aren't allowed to get on with that bit now. The misery is when they have to keep trying to attain something…

(Sonja, Carrie and Nadra, mixed mothers focus group, 2015)

What can be identified here is a shift in reproductive choices placed on women, through the dawn of reproductive technologies. Where the infertile previously had no choice, technology now *enables* a choice—it incites desire. This can be viewed as a pressure on women to become—or at least to try to become—mothers, for social acceptance and self-esteem. As highlighted by Gena Corea (1988) in her discussion of women's infertility before IVF, and which resonates with the above discussion:

> A few years earlier, a woman could, at some point, however painfully, come to terms with her infertility, go on with her life, find a way to live it fully. Now there is no easy way off the medical treadmill. She may now spend a major part of her adult life in debilitating treatment in experimental programs. There is always a promising new program to enrol in, its low success rate played down, it's "hope" played up. The years roll on. (1988, 3)

As Sonja explains, there are now many different ways to have a baby, whereas 'in previous times you'd just be childless'.

Through the discourse of choice, this exhibits a disciplinary power as it both incites a desire in the subject, but also, through the possibilities that reproductive technologies offer, administers a form of social control.

Not forcing women struggling with infertility to endure treatment, as passive victims, but, instead, inviting them to engage with it, in the pursuit of motherhood (Farquhar 1996; Petchesky 1987; Sawicki 1992). This opposes the argument by resistors (Lam 2015) collective Feminist International Network of Resistance to Reproductive and Genetic Engineering (FINNRAGE) who claimed that the development and commercialisation of assisted reproduction was exploiting women's bodies by turning them into machines—a form of violence against women (Corea 1985, 1988; Klein 1989; Rose 1994; Wajcman 1991). The main critique of this perspective is women were seen as the innocent and ignorant victims of men's conspiracy to take over their reproductive potential (Petchesky 1987; Throsby 2004).

However, through the focus groups' responses, it can be argued that these characters diagnosed with infertility are in fact *not* being represented as purely active agents, but reflect an element of the resistor's position, where childless women engaging with technological intervention are viewed as unwitting colluders in patriarchal control over women's bodies. Vulnerable women who have succumbed to the belief that to become a mother, through any means possible, is something, as Carrie stated, that they *must do*.

Therefore, this indeterminate tension of power discussed in the focus group data highlights how disciplinary power is the most useful tool to employ in this context. As Farquhar (1996) argues, reproductive technologies are neither evil nor good, that due to Foucault's belief that this form of power has a productive and transformation effect on the body, it can be viewed as both 'liberatory *and* controlling' (Farquhar 1996, 6). Controlling in the sense that, as Sonja stated: 'by hook or by crook you have to have it all', and liberatory due to there being so many 'different ways to have a baby'.

It has been proposed that the disciplinary practice of reproductive technologies aims to improve the infertile female body, as if the body were a machine to be fixed, rendering it more powerful, productive—more *reproductive*. This is enabled through the infertile woman becoming pregnant through IVF,[4] or for the surrogate to carry and deliver a genetic child for the intended parents. The end result is the same—normalising deviancy, fixing abnormalities, which is reflected in the narratives and character constructions in both *Giuliana & Bill* and *Coronation Street*. Both characters transition from non-mothers to mothers, from non-normative to normative, through the intervention of technologies, which mends their infertility. This notion of being fixed has also been identified by Karen Throsby (2004) in her work on IVF failure.

Throsby draws parallels between plastic surgery and IVF treatment, which she argues aims to modify and manage the body—to produce new bodies. Although the surrogacy process doesn't physically mend the woman's infertility, what it does do, through disciplinary medical intervention—for example, egg retrieval—is correct her position as a non-mother through the outsourcing of a fertile woman's womb. The abnormality of her *identity* is fixed through the acquisition of the genetic child—although in some cases donor eggs are also sourced—rescuing her from what I have argued is a deviant position outside of social norms. As Franklin argues: 'The inability to produce a biologically related child is represented in terms of a sense of exclusion, a lack of self-esteem or a loss of identity' (1990, 205). The heterosexual woman affected by infertility, like the lesbian—to be discussed in later chapters—is deemed as unfit for motherhood (Edge 2014). This can be applied to the representations of the characters disturbed by infertility in all of the texts under analysis, through the characters' expressions of unhappiness, and how divisions are created between the fertile (surrogate) and the infertile (intended mother) which 'subverts sisterhood' (Sandelowski 1990, 34).

Surrogacy as a non-normative practice is explored further in Chapter 4 through Shelley M. Park's (2006, 2014) discussion of how the adoptive maternal body is also positioned as defective, deviant, which she examines through the lens of queer theory. Park proposes that building families through adoption not only challenges traditional methods of procreation, through what Michael Warner (1993) describes as the goal of heterosexuality but deviates from the normative. The normative, she argues, drawing on a range of feminist work, is the naturalness of gestation, the genetic tie and genetic continuity—which resonates with Engel's claim that paternal lineage was of value as an assurance of female monogamy.

Although the majority of surrogacy cases share at least one genetic link to the child (which includes heterosexual *and* gay/lesbian couples)[5] I propose that the adoptive maternal body and the intended mother's maternal body share an affinity with same-sex parenthood, particularly homosexual men, as neither person carries the child. This can be identified in the separation of sex from reproduction—which also applies to lesbian couples—unless children exist from previous heterosexual relationships, *and* the removal from the gestational process, which is viewed as core to women's identity as mothers. As Park highlights, gestation and childbirth are considered a uniquely female experience, watching the body change and the foetus grow, which establishes an emotional connection, which she proposes is deemed only viable through biological motherhood.

As Giuliana says direct to camera, reflecting on her experience of watching the surrogate give birth: 'Watching Delphine push is pretty surreal. Of course, I wish I could have gone through this whole process myself, but I can't think about that right now'. Rose and Jess (pre-mothers focus group) identified with the value attached to carrying one's own pregnancy, by relating it to their own maternal aspirations. During a discussion of *Giuliana & Bill*, they shared their feelings of being 'really excited about being pregnant' (Rose) and 'I can't wait to have a bump' (Jess), both arguing that there must be a bond between the surrogate and baby as it is their body that is nurturing it and carrying it throughout its gestation. This reflects Charis Thompson's (2005) position that sharing a substance through gestation is more intimate than sharing genetics, being more 'uniquely characteristic of motherhood' (2005, 149–150).

Although this bond is made invisible in *Giuliana & Bill* through how the surrogate is positioned in the scenes—to be discussed in the following section—it drives the narrative in *Coronation Street*. The surrogate, Tina, bonds with baby Jake when she gives birth. As Laura (non-mothers focus group) points out: 'She [Tina] needed the money, but she changed from it being a completely financial process – a very cold, sort of matter of fact thing – to fuck! I love this baby! It totally switched from purely practical to totally emotional'. As Tina says to Izzy when she gives Jake back, after several high drama bust-ups: 'I fell in love with him when I held him, fed him. I knew he was your baby, but I thought he was mine, part of me'. Therefore, in addition, it can also be proposed that it is not just the intended mother who is positioned as non-normative through the process of surrogacy, but the surrogate also, as the gestation of a child of no genetic relation, to hand over at birth, can also be deemed as an abnormal maternal practice. Furthermore, drawing on Gorton's (2009) analysis of emotion in family-centred American TV drama *Brothers & Sisters*, what can also be identified through the construction of emotion in the narrative, as highlighted by Laura, is that outbursts of emotional expression are used as a vehicle for people to sort out their differences, 'however painful and however disparate' (2009, 135). This is seen in the emotional exchange between Tina and Izzy.

What can be identified further in the earlier exchange between Sonja, Carrie and Nadra (mixed mothers focus group) is a social pressure to conform to the conventional roles of motherhood. The way these participants discuss the construction of the characters infers that motherhood is obligatory, as something one *must do*. This suggests the assumption within compulsory heterosexuality that women *want* to have children, a sacred calling that is core to feminine identity (Rich 1980; Throsby 2004); a compulsory motherhood fuelled by the belief that the 'happy objects' of the baby and family will 'bring happiness to *us*' (Ahmed 2010, 26). This echoes the notion that, as Carrie detected through her reading of the texts, 'you're not valid if you don't have a child'.

As demonstrated in the work of Franklin (1990) which can be identified here, this pressure to produce a genetic child might result in emotional *and* physical stress. This is particularly true of IVF treatment as through its cyclical, treadmill-like nature and 'maybe next time promise' (Franklin 1997, 135) that the childless female subject finds detachment problematic. This nourishes the hopeful attachment of cruel optimism (Berlant 2011). This also applies to the surrogacy process, through embryo transfer. As Sonja pointed out: 'by hook or by crook you will have it all'. This can be read in the texts' final equilibrium of getting the baby, and drawing on Ahmed, the *ultimate* happy ending that gives life direction and purpose, enabling a 'happy heterosexuality' (Ahmed 2010, 90). This illuminates the belief that to *not* have it all, to *not* have the baby, positions the female subject as a failure, as the *loser*—located outside of the natural order. As Carrie identified, the possibility of building a childfree life is the part 'women aren't allowed to get on with', as the growth in options enabled by reproductive technologies means that women have no positive examples or guidelines to help them reorient onto the life path as non-mothers but are under pressure to 'keep trying' (Daniluk 1996; Throsby 2004).

Carrie's statement: '20 years ago it was like, oh, you can't have kids? That's such a shame, but there are a lot of other things you can do' also poignantly echoes Corea's (1988) position from this earlier period when she argued that 'a woman could, at some point, however painfully, come to terms with her infertility, go on with her life, find a way to live it fully. Now there is no easy way off the medical treadmill… There is always a promising new program to enroll in, its low success rate played down, its "hope" played up. The years roll on' (in Scutt 1990, 3). Drawing on Berlant (2008) and Franklin (1990, 1997), returning to the IVF treadmill with the desire to find a resolution through pregnancy is perpetuating the fantasy of normative family. Being in proximity to the object of desire preserves and refuels the desire for conventional family life, to belong to a larger world where motherhood and heterosexuality are the norm.

However, as Carrie explained, chasing this happy ending can also cause unhappiness, through continually 'trying to attain something' (read 'something' as the 'baby'). This anguished attachment to an idea of the good life/happy ending, which is wrapped up in the object of desire (the genetic baby), reflects Berlant's (2008, 2011) argument that the object that you *believe* will bring you happiness actually becomes the object that *destroys* your happiness. It's the presence of the possibility of happiness, which is enabled through the disciplinary practice of reproductive technologies ('you can do this, do this, or this'), which sustains cruel optimism.

Izzy (*Coronation Street*) and Giuliana (*Giuliana & Bill*) are depicted as the losers in the story, who need to be rehabilitated in order to fit in, as infertility has rendered them as objects of pity (Baraitser and Tyler 2010; Sandelowski 1993), and as unfit to parent (Edge 2014), until they *transition* into winners when their genetic babies are born. Izzy's situation evoked the most compassion from the focus groups participants. As Sally (mixed mothers focus group) stated: 'Out of all of their points of view, that was the one I thought, "Oh my god, what if I was in that situation?"' This demonstrates what cognitive film theorist Murray Smith (1995) describes as character engagement through the structure of sympathy, which he proposes occurs through an allegiance with the characters. In addition, Rebecca (non-mothers focus group) thought *Coronation Street's* surrogacy storyline was constructed with the most thought and detail: 'You got the most information about it all – the procedures *and* the feelings and emotions. It looked at it in a really sensitive way'.

In contrast, Giuliana and Bill as characters were evaluated by the participants as being false and self-obsessed. Rachel (non-mothers focus group) described the couple as 'horrible narcissists… it was so fake' as she argued their characters were performing for the audience, 'acting out' for the cameras (Kavka 2008, 97). Rachel and others in the focus groups felt that surrogacy in the show wasn't being taken seriously, a storyline employed purely for entertainment value. Ironically, in contrast to a genre named 'reality' TV, *Coronation Street* was viewed as more authentic, despite being fictional. However, due to the mechanism of melodrama that drives shows such as *Giuliana & Bill*, it is important to point out that the genre of reality TV and its relationship to *realism* are distant. As outlined by Peter Brooks (1996): 'the drive of realism is to understand the world by explaining it, whilst on the other hand melodrama forces meaning from the personal situations where language is inadequate and bodily gestures and somatic responses become the means by which the self is revealed' (in Skeggs and Wood 2012, 95).

Soap opera also employs melodrama, similarly to reality TV, for affective impact, alongside close-up angles for intimacy. However, the emotional connection with the focus group participants was noticeably stronger, primarily enabled through the multiple viewpoints. As Carrie (mixed mothers focus group) stated: 'It was more complex as it looked at it from every angle'. As freelance TV producer John Ellis (1999) explains: 'soap scenes open up major emotional questions to scrutiny… Soaps do so through the combination of empathy that accompanies narrative with a large degree of discussion of any one situation by the whole range of the soap's characters' (in Gorton 2009, 144).

It can be proposed, therefore, that the lack of multiple viewpoints in *Giuliana & Bill* has contributed to the audience perception of the show being 'fake', particularly in relation to the surrogate's representation, whose viewpoint appears to be blocked off, entirely. This will be returned to later on. Furthermore, it can also be proposed that the insincerity felt by participants could also be influenced by the docusoap style of reality TV, which *Giuliana & Bill* integrates into its format. As argued by Stella Bruzzi (2001), the key difference in this hybrid is that entertainment is prioritised over social commentary. Rachel (non-mothers focus group) in particular expressed her dislike to how before the episode of *Giuliana & Bill* had even finished, the E! channel (E! for entertainment) was already plugging the next show. Drawing on Jonathan Gray's (2010) work on television promos, this technique can be described as a '*textual* pull' which as he argues suggests that the '"text" for sale is the entire channel' (2010, 56–57). This she found extremely distasteful in the context of the sensitive topics of infertility and cancer that drive the show's narrative.

It is imperative to highlight here the significance of the differences between American and British contexts of the shows under discussion, specifically in relation to how the genre conventions differ within each territory. Despite family being central to both styles of soaps, key differences have been identified.[6] Not just through the distinctions of hi-gloss, excessive and lavish prime-time aesthetic versus raw realism (Crofts 1995; Geraghty 1991; Hollows 2012) but through how family melodrama and the maternal characters are shaped in the texts (Geraghty 1991). I return to this shortly.

Firstly, as mentioned earlier in this chapter, it is important to emphasise that British soap opera attempts to reflect working-class lives. At the time of writing, *Coronation Street* is Britain's longest-running soap opera. Based in Manchester and made by Granada Television, it was first transmitted on ITV in December 1960. *Coronation Street* has become symbolic of British working-class identity, primarily through its influence of social realism. Social realism in soap opera is when the daily lives of ordinary people are used to expose—or to understand and to explain (Brooks 1996)—current societal concerns. This provides, as argued by James Whittebols (2004), a 'window into the social mood of the time' (2004, 33). This is a primary function of British soaps, which I propose is influenced by the documentary's drive to represent current social issues and cultural values (Nichols 1991).

As highlighted by Christine Geraghty (1994) *Coronation Street* was created during a period of time when the creative fields of theatre, literature and cinema stressed the 'importance of drawing on different kinds of experience based on the lives of "ordinary people"' (in Allen 1994, 66). The arrival of *Coronation Street* marked an important cultural, social and political moment through its representation of a northern working-class community which featured strong and positive female characters (Feuer 1983).

This ambition to capture the social mood gives the genre, especially in long-term soaps such as *Coronation Street* and its BBC rival *EastEnders*, a more socio-realistic nature, based in family life and the community (Ang 1985; Carson and Llewellyn-Jones 2000; Geraghty 1991, 1994). As highlighted by Dorothy Hobson (2002), due to this focus, programmes such as these are able to express the interests of women, as she argues many of its characters are women facing similar issues, particularly in relation to themes of motherhood. Geraghty (1991) also claims that soaps validate the importance of female relationships and provide a space where emotional relationships are tested out. Feasey's (2017) work on maternal representations on TV, especially soap opera, also recognises motherhood as central to how the narrative is structured. She claims soaps, as well as reality TV and drama texts, are devoted to not the intensive mother, but the 'good enough' mother, 'mothers who love their children, cherish their families, but struggle with the financial, emotional, social or logistical reality of childcare' (2017, 7).

Geraghty proposes that family in British and American soaps are articulated differently. Not just through the British soap being more community-facing rather than being predominantly situated within the private home, as seen in *Dynasty* and *Dallas*, but through the positioning of and challenge to male authority. A useful perspective to employ here, in relation to the narratives of motherhood and family examined in this book, is Geraghty's extension of Laura Mulvey's (1989) distinction between the patriarchal and matriarchal melodrama. As Geraghty explains: 'Mulvey challenged the notion that fifties melodramas allowed a hidden or subversive expression of the problems and contradictions which underpin the construction of the family and the role of men and women within it' (1991, 61). Most importantly to Geraghty, however, is how Mulvey identified that in woman-dominated melodrama, the narrative is told from the woman's point of view. This is key in the discussion of soaps such as *Coronation Street*, particularly in light of how the participants in this study exhibited more empathy for its female characters than those portrayed in the other shows. As Geraghty points out: 'our knowledge is gained through her and we are invited to identify with her needs and dissatisfactions' (1991, 62). To explain the differences in how family is articulated in American and British soaps, Geraghty proposes that American soaps such as *Dallas* and *Dynasty* are patriarchal due to how the female characters refuse to be controlled by powerful men, whereas British soaps such as *Coronation Street* and *EastEnders* are matriarchal due to the male authority being bypassed by 'handing emotional and patriarchal control to the mother' (1991, 83). Geraghty claims that female viewers find both pleasurable.

Joanne Hollows (2012) has argued that was is interesting in Geraghty's analysis is how in British soaps matriarchs 'need not be biological mothers but can act as a mother to the community' (2012, 93). Therefore, the role of the mother in the British soap genre holds more social and cultural power than in its transatlantic counterpart. However, in relation to the analysis of the texts here, I challenge Geraghty's belief that soaps are built upon female solidarity, as in the context of the surrogacy storyline in *Coronation Street*, the female characters are being pitted against each other, and not united together, which is discussed further below. Despite this, the female participants in the focus groups were able to identify and empathise with *both* female protagonists—the intended mother (Izzy) and the surrogate (Tina)—due to the narrative technique of multiple viewpoints from primarily the woman's perspective.

Regardless of which character evoked the most sympathy from the focus group participants, both Izzy (*Coronation Street*) and Giuliana's (*Giuliana & Bill*) *loser* position is temporary, as they both eventually transform into *winners* when they become mothers, from a position of disappointment and desperation to one of fulfilment, where the fight against all odds results in a dream come true (Berlant 2008; Franklin 1990). However, although Giuliana's narrative journey is showered with disruptions, such as miscarriages and breast cancer, Izzy's transition into motherhood is depicted as more problematic. Not only did Izzy, like Giuliana, suffer loss through miscarriage, Tina decided to keep the baby after forming a bond at birth. As Izzy sobs to her partner Gary: 'He was my one and only chance. I don't want another baby. I just want Jake. She's got everything, and we've been left with nothing…' This shows the volatility of who is the winner and who is loser. It also demonstrates how the ideology of motherhood is shaped in the soap opera narrative. Maternal issues are the genre's driving force, this battle between the two women demonstrating how child-rearing is central—the mother figure being 'the heroine of the domestic text' (Geraghty 1991, 81). As Feasey (2013) claims: 'The soap opera does not merely represent motherhood, but rather it represents the "power of motherhood"' (2013, 32–33).[7] This helps to demonstrate how divisions are constructed between the women in the narrative through building tension based on difference and value attached to fertility, which 'defy female unity' (Sandelowski 1990, 34). This power of motherhood and central theme of maternal conflict is evident in all of the texts in focus for this project, across all genres, which have also been identified as key to the narratives that shape late-to-the-research-party dramas *The Handmaid's Tale* and *Top of the Lake: China Girl*. These shows will be discussed in Chapter 6.

While illustrating what has been described as a problematic and risky attachment to the object of desire, these examples also show the instability of the winner/loser binary that drives the narratives in both texts. I propose that these disruptions are simply narrative stepping-stones to the final equilibrium, and the goal, which is the acquisition of the genetic child. This is when the characters diagnosed with infertility transform into their new position. In the story, there can only be happy endings for some—unlike the loser, the winner takes it all (the genetic baby). Nevertheless, I propose that the loser in the story is not solely the childless character—until the happy ending is achieved. The loser is also reflected in the depictions of the surrogates, primarily through how they are framed and positioned on the screen in relation to the intended mothers. This, I argue, constructs what is a hierarchical division between the two bodies. Furthermore, through this exploration, the consideration of 'Other Mothers', particularly women of colour, emerges in relation to which bodies are allowed to be proximate to the object of desire, to transform, and those which aren't, to the point when they don't even make it into the frame, at all.

Out of the Frame

> I felt uncomfortable watching the first half of the clip as there wasn't a single image of the carrier at all, and I think the first thing they said was "gestational carrier". Then they cut to a clip where she was in the background, and the main focus was on the machine and readings – she was like a prop in the back of the scene. I thought it was horrible treatment of a woman that's gone out of her way to do that for someone else.
>
> (Charlie, non-mothers focus group, 2015)

The focus group participants commented on how the surrogate Delphine in *Giuliana & Bill* was positioned in the scenes, more than on any of the other surrogate representations that were discussed in the viewing sessions. Therefore *Giuliana & Bill* will provide the focus for this section, specifically the hospital scenes in 'Meet the Duke!' (Season 5, Episode 18) when the surrogate was in labour. The main reading by participants was that Delphine was rendered the most invisible, through how she was placed in the framing of the scenes, and how this silenced her point of view. I argue that these readings were influenced by the show's core genre conventions, which many of the participants were able to identify. Furthermore, I propose that through the participants' reflections hierarchies of power, status and privilege can be noted.

Charlie (non-mothers focus group) in particular took offence to Delphine's representation during the hospital scenes leading up the birth, as she felt that Delphine was being portrayed as a 'prop' in the background, seen as the holding vessel for the genetic child. Charlie also highlighted that 'gestational carrier', a term often used to describe Delphine, disturbed her. Gestational carrier is a name derived from legal documentation to describe a woman engaged in a commercial surrogacy arrangement, when a woman carries a child not genetically related to her for a fee. Such a description infers that Delphine is viewed by Giuliana as a carrier/object first, and a person/subject second. Charlie also found it discomforting that during Delphine's labour scenes an overexcited Giuliana adopting a doctor role dominated the scenes by pretended to read charts and order drugs, 'the main focus on the machine and readings'. This further illustrates the common thread of infertility narratives, which shows how the shift from conflict (infertility) to resolution (the baby) is enabled through medical terms and processes, which take over the story—the resolution being a medical cure (Franklin 1990). This is another example of how reality TV characters perform for the camera, to their audience (Kavka 2008).

As Rhian (pre-mothers focus group) stated: 'she [Giuliana] didn't seem emotional about the situation, she was more excited. She was like, doing it for the TV point of view'. This echoes Rachel's (non-mothers focus group) earlier assertion that Giuliana's hunger for a child was simply driven by a lifestyle commodity to be acquired, to show off to the camera and the wider world. Charlie's discomfort with how the surrogate has been represented sympathises further with the FINNRAGE position, who claimed that emerging practices such as commercial surrogacy were oppressive to women, as they signified men's control over women's bodies, for reproductive purposes. The resistors (Lam 2015) argued that surrogate bodies are seen as passive containers for reproduction, described as inanimate objects such as incubators, receptacles and vessels—maternal subjectivity erased, made invisible. As Rebecca (non-mothers focus group) expressed: 'It was very cold, with the 3D scan it was like they were treating her like an object'.

During Delphine's labour scenes, Bill is filming Giuliana. The dialogue exchanges occur interview-style from behind the camera. The introduction to the hospital scenes is framed through the use of a hand-held camera. Moving from a shot of the medical centre, the full screen is blacked out, which momentarily positions the viewer behind the camera. The red 'record' sign flashes in the corner. A close-up of Giuliana's face shows her removing the camera's lens cap: 'Oh wait, hold on, this isn't open'. As introduced earlier, the use of the hand-held camera demonstrates the influence of observational documentary's cinema verité, where the voice behind the camera creates a more situated and intimate presence (Nichols 1991). It has also been argued that the use of the hand-held camera embodies the human point-of-view, offering the viewer

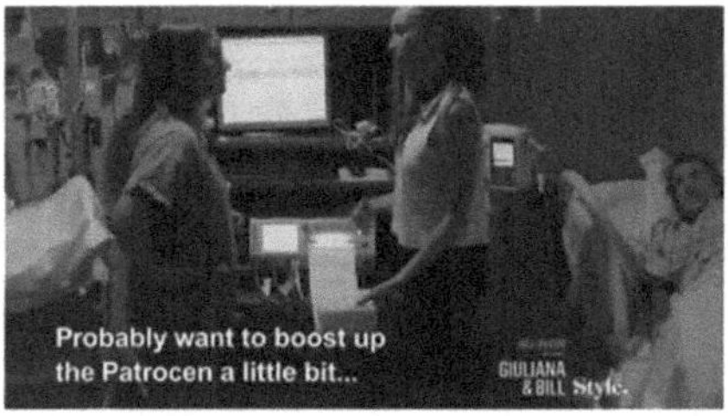

Fig. 2.3 *Giuliana & Bill*, Season 5, Episode 18, "Meet the Duke," Produced by Robert Sizemore, aired November 20, 2012 on E!, accessed July 21, 2017, E! 2009–2014, https://www.amazon.co.uk/gp/video/detail/B018YGPFEW?ref_=aiv_dp_season_select

a fly-on-the-wall perspective, which aims to capture moments as they unfold (Bruzzi 2001; Nash 2011).

During the filming of this scene, Giuliana has her back to Delphine (Fig. 2.3). There is little to no eye contact, and she barely speaks to her. Delphine remains silent, gazing up at Giuliana from the hospital bed. As Charlie described, Delphine is being portrayed as a 'prop'—an inanimate object, a foetal container. This scene also shows how pregnancy, particularly surrogate pregnancy, has become a managed process, which has shifted from a private to a public experience. In this instance, even more public by being shown on reality TV. Although the foetus itself is not in view, the 'machines' take a centre stage, which are in place to monitor foetal activity and the gestational carrier's labour. This illustrates how technology has been instrumental in the conceptual separation of the foetus from the maternal site, the advent and development of foetal imaging having constructed the foetus as a subject before its arrival, under the control and mediation of professionals.[8]

Delphine's marginalisation in these scenes shows how the foetus has eclipsed the maternal body from the central focal point (Duden 1993). As Charlie observed, the surrogate is positioned at the 'back of the scene'. This illustrates not only the transposition of personhood from the female subject onto the foetus, which in doing so forms the view of the surrogate body as merely a container, but what Carla Lam (2015) has identified as a new moment in reproductive technologies which alters the women's reproductive consciousness in relation to birth process—through not only the separation of sex from reproduction, but due to women being able to receive their genetic child 'without the labor of pregnancy and birthing' (2015, 33). As Paula (non-mothers focus group) highlighted, these intended mothers 'must feel the way a father must feel'. This masculine positioning in relation to how women diagnosed with infertility are constructed in the texts is explored further in Chapter 4.

Through Charlie's reading of the hospital scenes indicating a 'horrible treatment' of the surrogate, a hierarchical imbalance of power can be identified. This situates the surrogate, Delphine, as the loser in the narrative, through how she is positioned in the frame. It is important to highlight here that the 'frame' in this analysis can be viewed as symbolic, representing the frame of dominant heteronormative culture, the images and narratives that reside within it being constructed for the mainstream, heterosexual gaze (Cavalcante 2014; Dow 1996, 2001). The portrayal of the surrogate also unsettled Jess, Fay and Rose (pre-mothers focus group), particularly in the later scenes when Delphine was close to giving birth:

> Jess: There wasn't much about the baby in there, even when they were at the hospital you barely saw the woman who was giving birth, she was just in the corner of the screen.
> Fay: I thought they would've like, included the surrogate more seeing as it's about her surrogacy.
> Lulu: So, you thought she wasn't in it enough?
> Rose: You didn't see her point of view.
> Fay: I don't think she even spoke, did she?
> (Jess, Fay, Lulu, Rose, pre-mothers focus group, 2015)

This discussion further illustrates how the surrogate's maternal subjectivity has been erased, particularly through what appears to be the silencing of her character, due to being placed 'in the corner' of the screen which obstructs her perspective through the exclusion of dialogue. As Rose stated: 'You didn't see her point of view'. This underscores the polarities between the genre mechanisms of *Giuliana & Bill* and *Coronation Street*, where in the latter the multiple viewpoints evoked the most sympathy from the participants.

Delphine's silence during childbirth was also commented on. Rachel (non-mothers focus group) was convinced that sound had been deliberately edited out, and Nadra (mixed mothers focus group) thought that the silence was perhaps due to Scientology's mute birthing practice, despite no indication of the religion. Leading up to the baby's birth, Delphine is

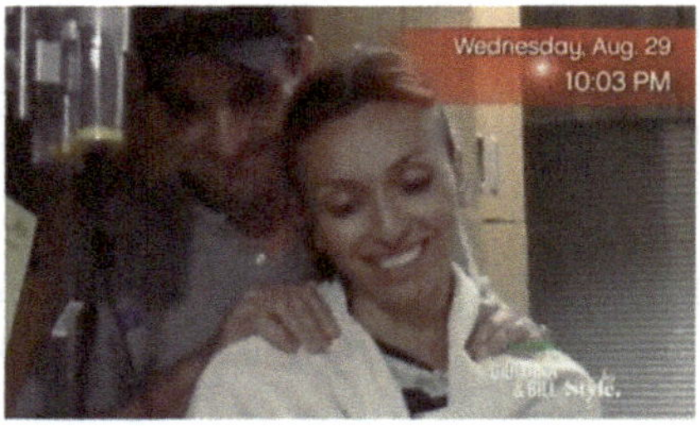

Fig. 2.4 *Giuliana & Bill*, Season 5, Episode 18, "Meet the Duke," Produced by Robert Sizemore, aired November 20, 2012 on E!, accessed July 21, 2017, E! 2009–2014, https://www.amazon.co.uk/gp/video/detail/B018YGPFEW?ref_=aiv_dp_season_select

continually edged out of the frame, just the top of her head remaining in view, while the camera locks on Giuliana's face, Bill standing behind her (Fig. 2.4). It could be suggested that this central positioning of Giuliana aims to strengthen her role as the genetic mother. Furthermore, it can be suggested the focus on Giuliana's face was engineered to capture her expressions leading up to the biggest money shot of all—the birth of her son. During their reflection of these scenes, Sonja and Carla (mixed mothers focus group) used words such as 'head' and 'dislocation' when discussing the surrogate's invisibility. This further marks the surrogate body as an object, a 'prop', which infers that the surrogate body is being represented, and read, as a machine for reproduction.

In her work on surrogacy and Marxism, Kelly Oliver (1989) argued that surrogacy provides a classic example of estranged labour, which she proposed exposes class and power imbalances. Marx believed that the worker is forced, by the drive for survival, to give his [sic] labour in the creation of commodities that 'produces for the rich wonderful things' (Marx 1844 in Lemert 2016, 34). Through the realisation of this labour, the worker finds himself losing a sense of the reality outside of himself, and a sense of himself. The estrangement, therefore, coming through the loss of the object he (in this context, 'she') is producing, which becomes alienated when it exists outside of him. Oliver's analysis centred on the hidden power imbalances in surrogacy contracts, proposing that the surrogate is working class or a minority, who provides her services, in exchange for money, for wealthy white middle-class women. Oliver argues that the sole purpose of the surrogate, like the worker in Marx's analysis, is to ‘produce and relinquish a flawless product no matter what physical and/or psychological pain she may suffer’ (1989, 106). Therefore, it is possible to argue that the rendering invisible of the surrogate through representation (or lack of) is also a method, aside from constructing her as an inanimate object and blocking her point of view, to silence any indication of her suffering, in order to produce a commodity.

Oliver claims that the language in the contracts masks inequalities by presenting the surrogate as an equal and autonomous agent. She believes that the surrogate’s freedom is merely an illusion. I argue that this masking of inequalities and illusion of autonomy is also evident in Giuliana’s relationship with the surrogate, Delphine, which has been read by the participants as manufactured and insincere. However, I propose that instead of the language in the surrogacy contracts, it is the use of emotion work, in the form of complements, which aims to disguise the imbalances of power. This is illustrated through one particular interaction with Delphine, when she is at the pushing stage of labour. Giuliana looks down at her and says: ‘Delphine, for what it’s worth you look really pretty. I swear to God, I’ve been thinking it all day!’ At this point Delphine is fully removed from the frame. Sonja and Nadra (mixed mothers focus group) thought calling her ‘pretty’ at this stage was condescending, inappropriate and an insincere expression of emotion, ‘so she would get the baby’. As Arlie Hochschild (2003) identifies in her work on the commercialisation of emotions: ‘Complementarity is a common mask for inequality in what is presumed to be owing between people’ (2003, 85). In the representation of Delphine throughout these scenes, any sign of her being an active subject was quashed by the dominance of Giuliana’s presence. However, as pointed out by Sonja (mixed mothers focus group) the genre mechanisms of the text contribute to the imbalance of power between Giuliana and Delphine:

> If they focused too much on the surrogate mum, they would risk losing the audience’s sympathy, and it’s all about portraying them as these great guys who’ve gone through a lot and still, you know… at the end it’s about seeing Giuliana and Bill with the baby.
>
> (Sonja, mixed mothers focus group, 2015)

Sonja’s comment resonates with the earlier discussion of how characters are constructed to engage emotionally with viewers, by evoking a sympathetic response. Once again, Sonja’s reading of the text demonstrates how these genre techniques have failed. The focus group participants found the show distasteful, most sympathy directed towards the surrogate and her depiction, rather than Giuliana's fertility journey—the antithesis to how the participants related to the intended mother, Izzy, in *Coronation Street*. Although some participants were sympathetic towards Giuliana's situation, her character was not received warmly. As Tara (non-mothers focus group) explained:

> For me it [*Giuliana & Bill*] encapsulated the notion of privilege and entitlement. At no point was it like, maybe this [motherhood] isn't for me. So yeah, she had gone through this amazing journey, but for a lot of people they would've just said, you know what, I can't afford to do this, it's not meant to be. So, it's privilege.
>
> (Tara, non-mothers focus group, 2015)

Although Tara didn't directly refer to race in her statement, what can be identified here is the proposition that reproductive technologies are only viewed as accessible to a specific category of user, which in the majority of these representations are white, educated, heterosexual married couples, such as Giuliana and Bill who have the benefits of white privilege. Although character Izzy in *Coronation Street* can be described as an 'Other Mother' due to her disability, she also benefits from white privilege, despite being working class. Izzy is also heterosexual and partnered at the time of the arrangement (they later break up). Therefore, this marks her as normative—she fits the ideal user category for assisted reproduction.

As has been argued by Dorothy Roberts (1995, 1996, 2000) the value of perpetuating the genetic line is to preserve racial purity, enabled through the disciplinary practice of reproductive technologies, which Roberts argues America, in particular, is obsessed with. This is evident in the absence of women of colour from representation in the texts explored in this chapter. Myths of the bond of the genetic tie will be explored in Chapter 5. Therefore, it can be proposed that through this exclusion, beliefs of racial purity are being reinforced, which reflects the dominant medical and media discourse that constructs infertility as white and heterosexual, technology made accessible to married, heterosexual couples. As aforementioned, Roberts claims that white women are shown as the primary consumers of reproductive technologies with images of 'white babies, usually with blond hair and blue eyes' (2009, 786). Roberts argues this through an IVF story in the *New York Times*

(1996) which pictures a fertility clinic director surrounded by seven white children, contrasted to news stories of accidental black babies born to white women through wrongly inseminated black sperm, 'intended to evoke revulsion precisely because of their race' (2009, 787). Throsby (2004) also highlights how images of the perfect mother and miracle child on TV and fertility clinics adverts are constructed as white and in heterosexual partnerships: 'the poster family for IVF' (2004, 2).

'Other Mothers' outside of this category of user are constructed as deviant, positioned outside heteronormative culture. However, this exclusion of women of colour, specifically, from the frame of assisted reproduction is ironic. According to experts in the field of race and reproductive technology, black women are one-and-a-half times more infertile than whites (Allen 1991; Arditti 1997; Briggs 2017; Farquhar 1996; Lam 2015; Roberts 1995, 2000). As Briggs (2017) highlights in her work on reproductive politics in America, in addition to this not only are African American women 'about half as likely to use ARTs' but they are also 'twice as likely as white women of matched economic class or age to lose a child in its first year of life, an epidemic of infant mortality increasingly documented by public health experts as an effect of racism' (2017, 16).

It can therefore be argued that cruel optimism and its objects of desire are more problematic, *more* risky, for some bodies than others—happy objects and the happy horizon placed out of reach. By rendering the black body invisible also points to Cathy J. Cohen's (1997) argument that black heterosexual bodies are excluded from dominant white heterosexual culture. This will be explored further in Chapter 5. Alongside the surrogates in these representations, it is the 'Other Mothers' that have been positioned as the real losers in the narrative, both in and out of the televisual frame.

Notes

1. This desperate baby hunger (Davitz 1984; Franklin 1990) can also be identified in TV drama *Top of the Lake: China Girl* (2017). The main storyline explores illegal transnational surrogacy arrangements between a number of infertile couples and Thai prostitutes in Sydney, Australia. All of the women are characterised much like the infertile female characters explored in this project—obsessive and emotionally unstable. In "Surrogate" (Season 2, Episode 3) one female character is presented as an extreme version of this. Once a successful concert pianist, she is shown wandering down a Sydney street mid-traffic in just her dressing gown, searching for her lost baby. As

her husband later explains to the police: 'She'd be okay if she had a baby, it would make her sane'. Not only does this position the heterosexual male on the more powerful side of the binary, as the voice of reason (woman/man, infertile/fertile, insane/sane) this also demonstrates Freud's notion that neurotic women can only be cured—normalised—by having a child, due to penis envy (Thompson 1943).

2. Briggs highlights the stark inequalities between American private insurance and Medicaid, which is the state health programme that provides coverage for the vulnerable (disabled, elderly, pregnant women) and those who are categorised as low-income. 'Private health insurers in more than ten states are required to provide infertility treatments to their employees, but none of those states provide it as a Medicaid benefit. Although the American Supreme Court has concluded that private employers need not cover employee's birth control, Medicaid mandates it – without a co-pay – and also covers sterilization' (2017, 108).
3. It is worth highlighting that although Giuliana is of Italian descent, as an Italian American she is categorised as white (Guglielmo and Salerno 2003). Therefore, for the purpose of this analysis, she is to be considered white.
4. It is important to note here that this discussion of IVF and surrogacy is reductive for focus, and that the processes can be far more complex—such as egg donation, egg donation *and* sperm donation, or three people IVF for mitochondrial disease prevention.
5. A favourable route for lesbian couples is to share biological motherhood through the gestational mother receiving a donor egg from her partner, through an IVF process called ROPA (Reception of Oocytes from Partner) (Fosas et al. 2010).
6. There has been debate over the definition of American and British soap operas, due to term being taken from the soap companies who targeted the female viewers of daytime American TV. However, despite the blurring of boundaries within the contexts and organisations such as the British Film Institute attempting to describe *Coronation Street* as serial drama, Geraghty (1991) argues that both American and British daytime shows are situated within the soap category. Not just due to daytime scheduling or appeal to female viewers, but 'the presence of stories which engage an audience in such a way that they become the subject of public interest' (1991, 4).
7. The last episode in *Top of the Lake: China Girl* is entitled 'Battle of the Mothers' (Season 2, Episode 6). As will be discussed in Chapter 6, this episode demonstrates how soap opera melodrama is now shaping contemporary TV dramas.
8. As discussed in Chapter 1, foetal imaging has contributed to the emergence of foetal personhood, which has influence film narratives. A more recent example of this in relation to the law can be seen in the morgue

scene in *Top of the Lake: China Girl*. In 'The Loved One' (Season 2, Episode 2), the coroner opens up the Thai prostitute's body to discover a 17–20 week-old foetus. He holds the foetus up to the light and says: 'Oh, it's a boy'. The case is then considered a double murder. However, according to the Supreme Court the current law in New South Wales, Australia, has a 'born alive rule'. This law would not consider the unborn child a second homicide as would not be viewed as a legally recognised person. This is not the only factual mistake this series makes in relation to the surrogacy storyline. Additional errors include inflating the financial recompense to surrogates in America and Australia by almost double.

References

Ahmed, Sara. 2006. *Queer Phenomenology: Orientations, Objects, Others*. London: Routledge.

Ahmed, Sara. 2010. *The Promise of Happiness*. Durham: Duke University Press.

Allen, Anita. 1991. "The Black Surrogate Mother." *Harvard BlackLetter Journal* (Spring): 17–31.

Ang, Ien. 1985. *Watching Dallas: Soap Opera and the Melodramatic Imagination*. New ed. London: Routledge.

Arditti, Rita. 1997. "Commercializing Motherhood." In *The Politics of Motherhood: Activist Voices from Left to Right*, edited by Alexis Jetter, Annelise Orleck, and Diana Taylor. Hanover, NH: University Press of New England.

Aslama, Minna, and Mervi Pantti. 2006. "Talking Alone: Reality TV, Emotions and Authenticity." *European Journal of Cultural Studies* 9 (2): 167–184.

Baraitser, Lisa, and Imogen Tyler. 2010. "Talking of Mothers." *Soundings: A Journal of Politics and Culture* 44 (1): 117–127.

Barrett, Michèle, and Mary McIntosh. 1991. *The Anti-Social Family*. New York: Verso.

Bell, Ann. 2010. "Beyond Financial Accessibility: Inequalities Within the Medicalisation of Infertility." *Sociology of Health and Illness* 32 (4): 631–646.

Benkov, Laura. 1994. *Reinventing the Family: The Emerging Story of Lesbian and Gay Parents*. New York: Crown Publishers.

Berlant, Lauren. 2008. *The Female Complaint*. Durham: Duke University Press.

Berlant, Lauren. 2011. *Cruel Optimism*. Durham: Duke University Press.

Borisoff, Deborah. 2005. "Transforming Motherhood: 'We've Come a Long Way,' Maybe." *Review of Communication* 5 (1): 1–11.

Braverman, Andrea Mechanick. 1997. "When Is Enough, Enough? Abandoning Medical Treatment for Infertility." In *Infertility: Psychological issues and counselling strategies*, edited by Sandra Leiblum. New York: Wiley.

Briggs, Laura. 2017. *How All Politics Became Reproductive Politics—From Welfare Reform to Foreclosure to Trump*. Berkley: University of California Press.

Brooks, Peter. 1996. *The Melodramatic Imagination*. New Haven: Yale University Press.
Brundson, Charlotte. 1997. *Screen Tastes: Soap Opera to Satellite Dishes*. London: Routledge.
Brundson, Charlotte. 2000. *The Feminist, the Housewife, and the Soap Opera*. Oxford: Oxford University Press.
Bruzzi, Stella. 2001. "Docusoaps." In *The Television Genre Book*, edited by Glenn Creeber, Toby Miller, and John Tulloch. London: BFI.
Carroll, Noel. 1990. *The Philosophy of Horror*. 1st ed. London: Routledge.
Carroll, Noel. 1996. *Theorizing the Moving Image*. Cambridge: Cambridge University Press.
Carroll, Noel. 2008. *On Criticism*. London: Routledge.
Carson, Bruce, and Margaret Llewellyn-Jones. 2000. *Frames and Fictions on Television: The Politics of Identity Within Drama*. Bristol: Intellect.
Cavalcante, André. 2014. "Anxious Displacements: The Representation of Gay Parenting on Modern Family and The New Normal and the Management of Cultural Anxiety." *Television & New Media* 1 (18): 454–471.
Ceballo, Rosario. 1999. "'The Only Black Woman Walking the Face of the Earth Who Cannot Have a Baby': Two Women's Stories." In *Women's Untold Stories: Breaking Silence, Talking Back, Voicing Complexity: Different Lives, Different Voices*, edited by Mary Romero and Abigail Stewart. New York: Routledge.
Charlebois, Justin. 2011. *Gender and the Construction of Hegemonic and Oppositional Femininities*. Lanham: Lexington.
Chodorow, Nancy. 1999. *The Reproduction of Mothering: Psychoanalysis and the Sociology of Gender*. Berkeley: University of California Press.
Cohen, Cathy J. 1997. "Punks, Bulldaggers, and Welfare Queens: The Radical Potential of Queer Politics?" *GLQ: A Journal of Lesbian and Gay Studies* 3 (4): 437–465.
Corea, Gena. 1985. *The Hidden Malpractice: How American Medicine Mistreats Women*. London: HarperCollins.
Corea, Gena. 1988. *The Mother Machine*. London: The Women's Press.
Coronation Street. 1960–present. Created by Tony Warren. TV programme. Manchester: ITV.
Couldry, Nick. 2002. *Media Rituals: A Critical Approach*. London: Routledge.
Crofts, Stephen. 1995. "Global Neighbours?" In *To Be Continued… Soap Operas Around the World*, edited by Robert C. Allen. London: Routledge.
Daniluk, Judith. 1996. "When Treatment Fails: The Transition to Biological Childlessness for Infertile Women." *Women in Therapy* 19 (2): 81–98.
Davitz, Lois. 1984. *Baby Hunger*. 1st ed. Minneapolis: Winston Press.
Dhoest, Alexander. 2005. "The Pfaffs Are Not Like the Osbournes: National Inflections of the Celebrity Docusoap." *Television and New Media* 6 (2): 224–245.

Dow, Bonnie. 1996. *Prime-Time Feminism: Television, Media Culture, and the Women's Movement Since 1970*. Philadelphia: University of Pennsylvania Press.
Dow, Bonnie. 2001. "Ellen, Television, and the Politics of Gay and Lesbian Visibility." *Critical Studies in Media Communication* 18 (2): 123–140.
Duden, Barbara. 1993. *Disembodying Women: Perspectives on Pregnancy and the Unborn*. Cambridge: Harvard University Press.
Edge, Brook Weihe. 2014. "Infertility on E! Assisted Reproductive Technologies and Reality Television." *Feminist Media Studies* 14 (5): 873–876.
El Nasser, Haya El, and Paul Overberg. 2007. "Fertility Rate on Upswing' USA Today. December 19, 2007. http://www.usatoday.com/news/nation/2007-12-19-fertility_N.htm.
Ellis, John. 1999. *Seeing Things: Television in the Age of Uncertainty*. London: I.B. Tauris.
Engels, Frederick. 2001. *The Origin of the Family, Private Property and the State*. London: Penguin.
Engwall, Kristina, and Helen Peterson. 2013. "Silent Bodies: Childfree Women's Gendered and Embodied Experiences." *European Journal of Women's Studies* 20 (4): 376–389.
Faludi, Susan. 1993. *Backlash: The Undeclared War Against Women*. London: Vintage.
Farquhar, Dion. 1996. *The Other Machine: Discourse and Reproductive Technologies*. London: Routledge.
Feasey, Rebecca. 2013. "From Soap Opera to Reality Programming: Examining Motherhood, Motherwork and the Maternal Role on Popular Television." *Imaginations: Journal of Cross-Cultural Image Studies* 4 (2): 25–46.
Feasey, Rebecca. 2015. *Mothers on Mothers: Maternal Readings of Popular Television*. Edinburgh: Edinburgh University Press.
Feasey, Rebecca. 2017. "Good, Bad or Just Good Enough: Representations of Motherhood and the Maternal Role on the Small Screen." *Studies in the Maternal* 9 (1): 5, 1–31, https://doi.org/10.16995/sim.234.
Feuer, Jane. 1983. "The Concept of Live Television: Ontology as Ideology." In *Regarding Television*, edited by Ann Kaplan. Frederick, MD: University Publications of America.
Finkelstein, Joanne. 1990. "Biomedicine and Technocratic Power." *Hastings Center Report* 20: 13–16, https://doi.org/10.2307/3562760.
Fosas, N., et al. 2010. Sharing Motherhood: Biological Lesbian Co-mothers, a New IVF Indication. *Human Reproduction* 25 (4): 938–941.
Foucault, Michel. 1977. *Discipline and Punish: The Birth of the Prison*. London: Penguin.
Franklin, Sarah. 1990. "Deconstructing Desperateness': The Social Construction of Infertility in Popular Representations of New Reproductive Technologies"

In *The New Reproductive Technologies*, edited by Maureen McNeil, London: Palgrave Macmillan.
Franklin, Sarah. 1997. *Embodied Progress: A Cultural Account of Assisted Conception*. London: Routledge.
Geraghty, Christine. 1991. *Women and Soap Opera: A Study of Prime Time Soaps*. Cambridge: Polity Press.
Geraghty, Christine. 1994. "Social Issues and Realist Soaps: A Study of British Soaps in the 1980s/1990s." In *To Be Continued… Soap Operas Around the World*, edited by Robert C. Allen. London: Routledge.
Giuliana & Bill. 2009–2014. "Meet The Duke." Season 5, Episode 18. Executive Producer Robert Sizemore. TV programme. November 20, 2012. Los Angeles, CA: E!.
Giuliana & Bill. 2009–2014. Executive Producers Alastair Surprise, Robert Sizemore. TV Programme. Los Angeles, California: E!
Gledhill, Christine. 1987. "Speculations on the Relationship Between Soap Opera and Melodrama." *Quarterly Review of Film and Video* 14 (1–2): 103–124.
Gorton, Kristyn. 2009. *Media Audiences*. Edinburgh: Edinburgh University Press.
Gray, John. 2010. "'Coming Up Next': Promos in the Future of Television and Television Studies." *Journal of Popular Film & Television Studies* 38 (2): 54–57.
Grindstaff, Laura. 2002. *The Money Shot: Trash, Class and the Making of TV Talk Shows*. Chicago: University of Chicago Press.
Guglielmo, Jennifer, and Salvatore Salerno. 2003. *Are Italians White?: How Race is Made in America*. New York: Routledge.
Hewlett, Sylvia Ann. 2002. *Baby Hunger: The New Battle for Motherhood*. London: Atlantic.
Hill, Annette. 2004. *Realty TV Audience and Popular Factual Television*. London: Routledge.
Hill Collins, Patricia. 2006 "Black Women and Motherhood." In *Motherhood and Space: Configurations of the Maternal through Politics, Home, and the Body*, edited by Caroline Weidmer, and Sarah Hardy. New York: Palgrave Macmillan.
Hirsch, Marianne. 1997. *Family Frames: Photography, Narrative, and Postmemory*. Cambridge: Harvard University Press.
Hobson, Dorothy. 1982. *Crossroads: Drama of a Soap Opera.*. London: Methuen.
Hobson, Dorothy. 2002. *Soap Opera*. Cambridge: Polity Press.
Hochschild, Arlie. 2003. *The Managed Heart. Commercialization of Human Feeling*. Anniversary edition. Berkeley: University of California Press.
Hollows, Joanne. 2012. *Feminism, Femininity and Popular Culture*. Manchester: Manchester University Press.
Kaplan, Anne. 1992. *Motherhood and Representation: The Mother in Popular Culture and Melodrama*. London: Routledge.
Kavka, Misha. 2008. *Reality Television, Affect and Intimacy*. Hampshire: Palgrave Macmillan.

Klein, Renate. 1989. *Infertility: Women Speak Out About Their Experiences of Reproductive Medicine*. Melbourne: Spinifex Press.
Lam, Carla. 2015. *New Reproductive Technologies and Disembodiment*. 1st ed. Abingdon: Routledge.
Lehr, Valerie. 1999. *Queer Family Values: Debunking the Myth of the Nuclear Family*. Philadelphia: Temple University Press.
Lemert, Charles. 2016. *Social Theory: The Multicultural, Global and Classic Readings*. 6th ed. Boulder: Westview Press.
Littler, Jo. 2013. "The Rise of the 'Yummy Mummy': Popular Conservatism and the Neoliberal Maternal in Contemporary British Culture." *Communication, Culture and Critique* 6 (2): 227–243. https://doi.org/10.1111/cccr.12010.
Mulvey, Laura. 1989. *Visual and Other Pleasures*. 1st ed. Bloomington, IN: Indiana University Press.
Mumford, Laura. 1991. "Plotting Paternity: Looking for Dad on Daytime Soaps." *Genders* 12: 45–61.
Mumford, Laura. 1995. *Love and Ideology in the Afternoon: Soap Opera, Women, and Television Genre*. Bloomington: Indiana University Press.
Nash, Kate. 2011. "Documentary-for-the-Other: Relationships, Ethics and (Observational) Documentary." *Journal of Mass Media Ethics* 26: 224–239.
Nelson, Fiona. 2007. "Mother Tongues: The Discursive Journeys of Lesbian and Heterosexual Women into Motherhood." *Journal of GLBT Family Studies* 3: 223–265.
Nelson, Fiona. 2009. *In the Other Room: Entering the Culture of Motherhood*. Nova Scotia, Canada: Fernwood Publishing.
Nichols, Bill. 1983. "Myth and Narrative in Documentary." *Film Quarterly* 41 (1): 9–20.
Nichols, Bill. 1991. *Representing Reality*. Bloomington, IN: Indiana University Press.
O'Donohoe, Stephanie. 2006. "Yummy Mummies: The Clamor of Glamour in Advertising to Mother." *Advertising & Society Review* 7 (3): 1–21.
Oliver, Kelly. 1989. "Marxism and Surrogacy." *Ethics & Reproduction* 4 (3): 95–115.
Park, Shelley M. 2006. "Adoptive Maternal Bodies: A Queer Paradigm for Rethinking Mothering?" *Hypatia* 21 (1): 201–226.
Park, Shelley. 2014. *Mothering Queerly, Queering Motherhood*. New York: State University of New York Press.
Petchesky, Rosalind. 1987. "The Power of Visual Culture and the Politics of Reproduction." *Feminist Studies* 13 (2): 263–292.
Rich, Adrienne. 1980. "Compulsory Heterosexuality and Lesbian Existence." *Signs: Journal of Women in Culture and Society* 5 (4): 631–660.
Roberts, Dorothy. 1995. "The Genetic Tie." *The University of Chicago Law Review* 62 (1): 209–273.

Roberts, Dorothy. 1996. "Race and the New Reproduction." *Faculty Scholarship at Penn Law.* 1154.

Roberts, Dorothy. 2000. *Killing the Black Body: Race, Reproduction, and the Meaning of Liberty.* New York: Vintage Books.

Roberts, Dorothy. 2009. "Race, Gender, and Genetic Technologies: A New Reproductive Dystopia?" *Signs: Journal of Women in Culture and Society* 34 (4): 783–804.

Rose, Hilary. 1994. *Love, Power and Knowledge: Towards a Feminist Transformation of the Sciences.* Cambridge: Polity Press.

Rose, Gillian. 2010. *Doing Family Photography: The Domestic, The Public and the Politics of Sentiment.* London: Routledge.

Katz Rothman, Barbara. 2000. *Recreating Motherhood.* 2nd ed. New Brunswick, NJ: Rutgers University Press.

Rules of Engagement. 2007–2013. Created by Tom Hertz. TV Programme. New York: CBS.

Sandelowski, Margarete. 1990. "Fault Lines: Infertility and Imperiled Sisterhood." *Feminist Studies* 16 (1): 33.

Sandelowski, Margarete, and Sheryl de Lacy. 2002. "The Uses of 'Disease': Infertility as a Rhetorical Device." In *Infertility Around the Globe: New Thinking on Childlessness, Gender and Reproductive Technologies*, edited by Marcia Inhorn and Frank van Balen. Berkeley: University of California Press.

Sawicki, Julia. 1992. *Disciplining Foucault: Feminism, Power, and the Body.* New York: Routledge.

Schickel, Richard. 2000. *Intimate Strangers: The Culture of Celebrity in America.* Lanham, MD: Ivan R Dee, Inc.

Scutt, Joceyln. 1990. *The Baby Machine: Reproductive Technology and the Commercialisation of Motherhood.* London: Merlin Press.

Skeggs, Beverley, and Helen Wood. 2012. *Reacting to Reality Television, Performance, Audience and Value.* Oxon: Routledge.

Smith, Murray. 1995. *Engaging Characters: Fiction, Emotion and the Cinema.* Oxford: Clarendon Press.

Smith, Gregg. 1999. "Local Emotions, Global Moods and Film Structure." In *Passionate Views: Film, Cognition, and Emotion*, edited by Carl Plantinga and Greg Smith. Baltimore: John Hopkins University Press.

Smith, Gregg. 2008. *Film Structure and the Emotion System.* Cambridge: Cambridge University Press.

Spencer, Amy. 2012. "Giuliana Rancic: How I Got Through the Tough Stuff." *Health*, November 20. http://www.health.com/health/article/0,,20637654,00.html.

Taylor, Janelle. 1992. "The Public Fetus and the Family Car: From Abortion Politics to a Volvo Advertisement." *Public Culture* 4 (2): 67–80.

The New Normal. 2012–2013. TV Programme. Created by Elodie Keene, Max Winkler, Ryan Murphy. New York: NBC.

Thompson, Clara. 1943. "'Penis Envy' in Women." *Psychiatry, Interpersonal and Biological Processes* 6 (2): 123–125.

Thompson, Charis. 2005. *Making Parents: The Ontological Choreography of Reproductive Technologies.* Cambridge, MA: MIT Press.

Throsby, Karen. 2004. *When IVF Fails. Feminism, Infertility and the Negotiation of Normal.* Basingstoke: Palgrave.

Tincknell, Estella. 2005. *Mediating the Family: Gender, Culture and Representation.* London: Bloomsbury.

Todorov, Tzvetan. 1990. *Genres in Discourse.* Cambridge: Cambridge University Press.

Top of the Lake: China Girl. 2017. "Surrogate". Season 2. Episode 3. Directed by Ariel Kleiman. Written by Jane Campion and Gerard Lee. TV programme. May 23, 2017. New York: Sundance BBC.

Wacjman, Judy. 1991. *Feminism Confronts Technology.* Cambridge: Polity Press.

Warner, Michael. 1993. *Fear of a Queer Planet: Queer Politics and Social Theory.* Minneapolis: University of Minnesota Press.

Whittebols, James. 2004. *The Soap Opera Paradigm: Television Programming and Corporate Priorties.* Lanham, MD: Rowman and Littlefield.

Williams, Linda. 1984. "'Something Else besides a Mother': 'Stella Dallas' and the Maternal Melodrama." *Cinema Journal* 24 (1): 2–27.

Williams, Linda. 1991. "Film Bodies: Gender, Genre, and Excess." *Film Quarterly* 44 (4): 2–13.

CHAPTER 3

Becoming Ordinary: Making Homosexuality More Palatable

This chapter explores the representations of homosexual and lesbian characters in relation to the surrogacy plotline in two American sitcoms, *The New Normal* and *Rules of Engagement*. *The New Normal* follows the journey of homosexual couple Bryan and David as they build a family through surrogacy, and in *Rules of Engagement* lead heterosexual couple Audrey and Jeff engage their lesbian friend Brenda to be their surrogate.

This chapter's primary argument is that through the narrative vehicle of surrogacy, and the employment of the conventional sitcom formula, the homosexual characters in *The New Normal* have been constructed to present a specific type of homosexuality which is more palatable to mainstream audiences—white, affluent, masculine and situated within a monogamous, loving relationship.

In the analysis of the lesbian surrogate in *Rules of Engagement*, what will be of focus is how the character's masculine traits transform to become more conventionally feminine through the pregnancy process, which results in the lesbian being depicted as becoming more of a woman from a previous non-woman masculine position. This, I argue, reflects Monique Wittig's (1992) claim that 'lesbians are not women' (1992, 57) due to lesbianism as a concept not being wholly recognised ideologically, socially, legally or politically within heterosexual culture. Furthermore, the butch–femme model that originated in lesbian culture, in relation to the construction of femininity and masculinity within the couple dyad, will also be evoked to explore the positioning of the

L. Le Vay, *Surrogacy and the Reproduction of Normative Family on TV*, Palgrave Studies in Science and Popular Culture,
https://doi.org/10.1007/978-3-030-17570-2_3

homosexual characters, in relation to what is, and what isn't, deemed acceptable in relation to same-sex parenting. Butchness in relation to the lesbian character will be explored through the transition from masculine to feminine traits, through pregnancy.

To explore how the raced and gendered sexualities of the characters have been constructed within the texts, I employ the concept *queer straightness*, which I have devised to describe how the creation of family through surrogacy, and the process of pregnancy, aims to make the gay characters more palatable to mainstream audiences. This, as I propose, is enabled through the narrative's 'happiness scripts', which 'can be thought of as straightening devices' (Ahmed 2010, 91). Through these devices, I argue that the gay characters are realigned in the normative; positioned in proximity to signs of happiness—and therefore signs of straightness—such as the reproduction of genetic children, women's experience of pregnancy, the family home and the couple dyad (Ahmed 2006, 2010). As Ahmed (2010) claims, these signs are symbolic of the straight line of normative heterosexuality: 'ways of aligning bodies with what is already lined up' (2010, 91). I propose that the *queer straightness* that shapes the texts' narratives does so to situate the characters as socially accepted, happy and *normalised*. These characters are constructed to embody a category of homosexuality that is recognised and deemed appropriate by mainstream popular culture, to a 'world that has already decided what *is* acceptable' (2010, 106).

Furthermore, what will also be explored is how the deviancy of same-sex sexual intimacy has been disciplined through the love plot, which not only steers the monogamous relationship of the homosexual couple in *The New Normal*, but also, in *Rules of Engagement*, is central to the narrative of the lesbian body carrying a child to support heterosexual love and reproduction. I argue that normative sexuality is inferred, through which narratives of sentimentality, romance and domesticity materialise, which are rooted in late nineteenth- and early twentieth-century ideologies of family. In addition, the desire to create a family in the reflection of normative heterosexuality will also be discussed.

Through dialogic textual-audience analysis, I argue that the representations articulate a good homosexuality, which not only aims to construct the 'normal gay' (Seidman, 2004, 14) but also obscures explicit sexual intimacy between same-sex couples, beyond hand holding and a peck on the mouth. Therefore, the family home, as a sign of straightness (Ahmed 2010), which are central settings to both texts, signifies that the love for a *future foetus*, and the *future family*, eclipses the romantic love narrative. Becoming parents not only rescues the characters from deviancy, but resolves, or placates, anxieties of homosexual intimacy and the threat that same-sex desire may endanger the genetic line of descent. The way the gay characters have been presented in both *The New Normal* and *Rules of Engagement* suggests that mainstream popular culture *only* accepts homosexuality and lesbianism if it is packaged in a more heteronormative form.

Sitcom conventions and the use of comedy as a form of social and cultural power will also be addressed, with a particular focus on the use of the stereotype, in relation to how ideologies of race, gender and family are shaped in the texts. The concept of *queer straightness* will also underpin a discussion on how the construction and depiction of same-sex partnerships and the creation of family both challenge and reproduce heterosexual norms of the nuclear family. The concept of *queer straightness* will be unpacked in this chapter by drawing on a range of queer and feminist work on homosexual and lesbian experience and media representation, queer families, heteronormativity and emotions and affect.

This chapter unfolds over three sections. "Just Your (Stereo)type" explores the representation of homosexuals and same-sex parenting, with a focus on the use of the stereotype and humour as its key genre device. "Crying Like a Girl" examines the representation of lesbianism in the context of pregnancy, motherhood and conventional notions of hetero-femininity, and "Fitting In" will show how the characters' sexual identity is disciplined to become more acceptable through being situated within a heteronormative narrative framework.

Just Your (Stereo)type

> They're obviously making a programme about gay people as there aren't enough. But then they're making it really stereotypical.
>
> (Rose, pre-mothers focus group, 2015)

Rose (pre-mothers focus group), who was responding to clips from *The New Normal*, pinpointed the fact that there are still very few representations of 'gay people' on fictional TV when compared to the saturation of heterosexual representation across popular media. However, TV shows, specifically sitcoms that feature gay characters are continuing to grow. According to the latest report by American LGBTQ media monitoring organisation GLAAD (2018), who have been tracking the presence of lesbian, gay, bisexual, transgender and queer characters on television since 1995, the numbers are on the increase. The 2018 study reported an increase of almost double from the previous year, the quantity of LGBTQ characters being represented across scripted prime-time television climbing from 4.8 to 8.8%. Another significant change that has been noted is that for the first time the gender parity of the characters is equal, whereas previously the majority of this LGBTQ representation belonged to white homosexual men.

Further shifts include Netflix women-in-prison show *Orange Is the New Black* (2013–present) which features the largest proportion of leading lesbian, transgendered and bisexual characters in a series. GLAAD and Harris Poll's *Accelerating Acceptance* study (2018) also revealed that a substantial 20% of Americans aged 18–34 identify as LGBTQ. This finding is key for networks moving forward. However, as President and CEO of GLAAD Sarah Kate Ellis states, it's not about box ticking character inclusion, these representations have to be authentic to connect with the LGBTQ audience. As she argues: 'there needs to be nuance and depth to their story and they should reflect the full diversity of our community' (WWAOTV 2018).

The first lead openly gay character who appeared on prime-time American sitcom in 1998, was Will Truman in hit show *Will & Grace* (1998–2006, 2017–present). Since then, homosexual characters have appeared in numerous popular prime-time shows including *Sex and the City* (1998–2004), *My So-Called Life* (1994–1995), *Glee* (2009–2014), *True Blood* (2008–2014), *Ugly Betty* (2006–2010), and *The Simpsons* (1989–present). However, the representation of same-sex characters in the context of building a family is still relatively new. Aside from representations in films such as lesbian family flick *The Kids Are All Right* (2010) and the passing-as-straight closet movie *The Birdcage* (1996), television representations are sparse, with same-sex parented families having only emerged in TV dramas such as hospital hit *Grey's Anatomy* (2005–present), family shows *The Fosters* (2013–present) and *Brothers & Sisters* (2006–2011), and in sitcoms *Modern Family* (2009–present) and *The New Normal* (2012–2013). The homosexual characters in *Brothers and Sisters* and *Modern Family* create families through adoption. In addition to the adoption storyline, *Brothers & Sisters* also features a surrogacy storyline, which appears in the final season. *The New Normal* was cancelled after one season. This was due to a drop in the ratings, which Christian campaigners OneMillionMoms.com, a division of the American Family Association, claim was the result of their ardent campaigning against the show's narrative. They believed the show promoted a decline in social values and morals by aiming to redefine marriage and family structures (Queer Voices 2016). *The New Normal* is the only prime-time show to feature two lead homosexual characters in a committed and monogamous relationship, with a surrogacy storyline at its centre.

As Rose stated, she thought that the representations of homosexuality in *The New Normal* were 'really stereotypical'. Therefore, the sitcom convention of the stereotype, and the use of humour, will provide the focus for this section. I argue these genre conventions frame a range of ideologies in the texts, shaping ideals of family, sexuality, race and gender. Furthermore, although *The New Normal* is of key focus, references to—and analyses of—other sitcoms such as *Modern Family* and *Will & Grace* will be referred to, to support the argument.

The analysis of the audience data revealed both positive and negative readings of how the homosexual couple is represented. Both positions will be examined. However, what is important to highlight at this juncture is that the focus group participants detected more negative representations of the key lesbian character Brenda in *Rules of Engagement*, also referencing the minor lesbian characters in *The New Normal*. This will be treated separately in the following section.

The classic sitcom structure encompasses a recurring cast of characters based around the family unit, who perform within a 20–30-minute time slot. Although *The New Normal* appears progressive by depicting a same-sex couple creating a family through the non-conventional route of surrogacy, the core narrative framework is built on 1950s' sitcoms, which focus on the traditional family unit. The show also borrows from the later formation of family that consists of unrelated adults,[1] such as hit shows *Cheers* (1982–1993) and *Friends* (1994–2004).[2]

The central cast of characters in *The New Normal* includes the homosexual couple (David and Bryan), the gestational surrogate (Goldie), Goldie's grandmother (Jane, or 'Nana'), the surrogate's daughter (Shania) and Bryan's personal assistant (Rocky). This set of characters updates the traditional sitcom formula of blundering dad, queen-of-the-nest mother, cheeky boy and bubbly girl, and best friend (Mills 2005). However, I argue that this set of characters, with a specific focus on the central father/mother formula as it reappears in the construction of the two gay characters as soon-to-be-parents, situates them as normative by positioning the rest of the cast as non-normative. Bryan and David are white, educated, wealthy men in a monogamous long-term relationship. David is a gynaecologist, Bryan a TV writer. They share a beautiful home in an LA suburb. In contrast, the surrogate, Goldie, is positioned as working-class and financially desperate, which drives her to surrogacy.

Hailing from the Midwest, Goldie displays the region's characteristics, shown to lack 'the kind of sophistication, culture, and cosmopolitanism that define Bryan and David's lifestyle' (Cavalcante 2014, 8). Her grandmother Nana is offensive and disapproving. She hurls hyperbolic racist and homophobic slurs in almost every scene to every character, with lines such as: 'lesbians look like ugly men', 'what are you doing helping these salami smokers?' and 'I feel like I just woke up and ate some black and gay stew!' (Season 1, Episode 1: 'Pilot'). Rocky, Bryan's personal assistant (the black character) is African American and marked by racial stereotypes. Rocky is characterised as loud, abrasive, is prone to stealing, lying and is incapable of moving her career beyond being an assistant. When Bryan promotes her to TV producer at his company, she fails (Season 1, Episode 13: 'Stay-At-Home Dad'). Rhian, Rose and Fay (pre-mothers focus group) interpreted the representations of the homosexual characters in *The New Normal* as positive, in the context of the supporting characters:

Rhian: At least it's not negative.
Rose: Yeah, true, it's not.
Lulu: You don't think it's negative in any way?
Rhian: I think because that… what was her name, Nana, was represented as an evil person. Whatever she says is wrong. So, they're not represented negatively.
Fay: She *is* wrong, but she generates a laugh out of the pure shock of what she's just said. It's like, "wow, I can't believe it!" which makes you think it's wrongful what she's just said. It's rather the shock factor than "wow, that's so funny!"
(Rhian, Rose, Lulu and Fay, pre-mothers focus group, 2015)

André Cavalcante (2014) describes this as 'anxious displacements' (2014, 456). This is when 'the dynamics of anxiety and symbolic excess are projected away from LGBTQ characters onto those in their orbit' (2014, 3). In his analysis of both Bryan and David in *The New Normal*—and also Mitch and Cam in *Modern Family*, who adopt a child—he claims that these representations are shown as positive in the way that the cultural anxiety of same-sex parenting, and homosexuality in general, is averted away from the queer bodies and projected onto the other characters. The recipients of these anxious displacements, outside of the main cast of characters, include Shania's (the surrogate's daughter) school friend Wilbur, who is part Latino, and his promiscuously portrayed white single mother who doesn't know who his father is. This minor character is significant as she embodies traces of the white trash stereotype by indicating a class disgust through being poor and having a mixed-race child (Tyler 2008). The surrogate Goldie is also shaped through this stereotype by being white, working-class *and* a teen mother, who is driven to surrogacy to earn money so she can support her child. This therefore positions her in the narrative as irresponsible and incompetent: a bad mother (Feasey 2017; SmithBattle 2013). A discussion of the socio-economic positioning of the surrogates in *The New Normal* and *Baby Mama* are discussed in the following chapter.

Shania's Latino pal Wilbur is also presented as promiscuous. He is reprimanded for making inappropriate sexual advances to Shania (they are both 9-years-old). Alongside the depiction of the slutty single mother, the stereotypes of the supporting characters reflect sitcom's genre convention of mocking vulnerable groups. Brett Mills (2009) has identified a number of these groups—the coon, the lecherous Italian and the battle-axe mother-in-law, who he claims appear frequently on sitcom line-ups. In *The New Normal*, these stereotypes are constructed through Rocky (the coon), Wilbur (the lecherous Italian) and Nana (the battle-axe mother-in-law), who Rhian described as the 'evil one'. Calvacante argues that Nana is positioned in the narrative to receive the most anxious displacement by being painted as a relic of the past through her extreme bigotry. She was also the key supporting character that Rhian, Rose and Fay commented on. However, I propose that the construction of Nana's character is inserted into the narrative as a deflective device. Through the use of humour to provoke audience's laughs, she performs as a narrative decoy by distracting viewers to *not* read what I believe to be more serious racist and misogynistic undertones in relation to how the gay couple is shaped in the text. Rose (pre-mothers focus group) shared her concerns of racial stereotyping in popular media:

> I was speaking to my teacher the other day, and she was basically saying how she finds it difficult to find films that have black people playing a main serious role, and a lot of the time black people are played as, in a comedic way, so people can just laugh at them. I think some gay people probably

> would be offended that they were just put in a comedy, rather than a drama – a show with a serious side.
>
> (Rose, pre-mothers focus group, 2015)

Through a discussion of racial representation through the stereotype, Rose was able to recognise similar issues of how gay characters are represented, demonstrating a comparison between minority groups that has been widely documented (Fejes and Petrich 2013; Lucas and Raley 2006; Moritz 1987, 1999). Although Rose didn't provide a more nuanced reading of race in her reflections of *The New Normal*, she was able to hint towards deeper textual issues of dominant ideologies of power and race. For example, her statement 'so people can laugh at them' reflects concerns of how black characters have been represented on screen since the 1920s. Donald Bogle (2016) argues that the early character types of 'the coon, the tragic mulatto, the mammy and the brutal black buck' were stereotypes constructed to 'stress inferiority' (2016, 4). This was done, Bogle claims, through poking fun out of them. Terry Jones and Robert Staples (1985) highlight how concerns shifted from first getting blacks on the screen, to how they were depicted. Despite the increase in visibility throughout the 1980s, they argue that: 'the people who control what is shown on TV seem to believe that whites feel most comfortable with blacks playing the roles of fools, maids clowns, funny men and small time hustlers' (1985, 10). This claim can be identified in the portrayal of the African American female character Rocky in *The New Normal.* One scene in particular demonstrates this (Season 1, Episode 19: 'Blood, Sweat and Fears') where Rocky struggles to look after her newly adopted baby daughter, Nikki.

Rocky becomes flustered over getting Nikki dressed, and is unsuccessful in braiding what is shown as unruly black hair. The surrogate's young daughter Shania takes over child-care and shows Rocky how to be a mother, not only through her calm caretaking skills but also her improbable expertise in black hair management. The symbolism of this scene is striking. In her work on race and adoption, Katz Rothman (2005) claims that for white adoptive mothers of black children (as she herself experienced), the fixing of unruly black hair is political. It is a test that one passes or fails, as well as a sign of taming—representing slavery—and is of curiosity to white people. Black hair, Rothman argues, is 'loaded with meaning' (2005, 207).

This inability to manage her adopted daughter's hair therefore positions Rocky as a failed mother, a common representation of black motherhood in popular culture, especially when constructed as a black single mother. As Adrienne McCormick (2010) highlights: '… when we see black mothers who are not "moral compasses," they fail to balance motherhood, work, and sexuality – as the white mothers do – and are more likely to appear as failed mothers than as supermothers' (2010, 149). By swooping into rescue Rocky from being a bad mother, I argue Shania not only embodies this notion of the white 'supermother', but through this act of rescue is also symbolic of the white saviour narrative, a trope that has also been identified in *Modern Family*, through the white homosexual couple adopting a child from Vietnam (Cavalcante 2014).

Furthermore, Bryan, as Rocky's boss, provides her with an income, and inspires her to become a parent, too, albeit not a *real* one. Building a family through adoption is seen as outside of normative white family discourse (Park 2006, 2014). In addition, drawing on Briggs (2017) and Dána-Ain Davis' (2009) discussion of race and reproductive politics in America, I argue that Rocky is not able to achieve normative maternal status due to America's cultural and political logic that believes that 'women marked as being of color, poor or low income women, and single women do not have fertility problems that should be addressed' (in Briggs 2017, 109). Rocky's (possible) infertility is not spoken of in the narrative, and access to assisted fertility treatment, or commercial surrogacy services, is not considered. However, despite this, Rocky adopting an African American child ally with two important things: that there are a much larger proportion of African American children in the care system awaiting adoption, and that blood ties within black communities are deemed less important in the creation of families than they are in white America (Roberts 1996). Extended kinship structures will be explored in Chapter 5.

Rocky's subordinated relationship with Bryan, her adoption of a child, alongside both men's relationships with the surrogate, Goldie, constructs idealised images of white Americans (Hughey 2014), which further signifies white privilege. This emphasises, in the context of race and reproductive technologies, who has access to assisted reproduction, and who doesn't, and who is allowed into the representational frame, and who isn't. Both are core threads throughout this project. As Sara Ahmed (2010) identifies: 'Black and working-class women are not even entitled to be proximate to the fantasy, though they may be instrumental in enabling others to approximate its form' (2010, 51).

With Rose's sympathy towards the gay characters, and Rhian and Fay interpreting Nana's polemical outbursts as 'wrong' and 'evil', the portrayal of the central gay characters in their quest to build a family through surrogacy has been positioned predominantly positively. During the viewing sessions of *The New Normal*, the majority of the participants in the focus groups, including the lesbians, giggled at Nana's tirades. As Fay identified, the character 'generated a laugh out of pure shock'. This appeared to be unsettling for her, as she detected a tension between how it feels to laugh out of 'pure shock' or because something is funny. As Mills (2005) explains: 'viewers have yet to discover *how* they're meant to laugh at blacks, females or gays in contemporary comedy without inadvertently supporting power structures which keep these groups subordinated' (2005, 148).

I propose this generation of shock demonstrates how emotions are constructed in the narrative, through the sequence of scenes, dialogue and characterisation, which connects with the viewers to the point where certain emotions can literally be yanked out of them (Gorton 2009; Williams 1991). Linda Williams describes this method as 'jerking', in relation to melodrama and horror genres, but which can be applied here. She employs this term to explain how the audience is manipulated, though 'an over-involvement in sensation and emotion' (1991, 5). Where Williams talks about tear jerkers or fear jerkers, the participants' reaction to Nana's extreme outbursts could be described as shock jerkers—the stifled giggles indicating feelings of shame. However, it is important to note that this response could also have been the result of being situated in the more unnatural viewing experience of a focus group, away from a more relaxed and private home environment.

The shock-induced giggles, which spread within the groups, might be described as the contagion of affect, to incite shock (Ahmed 2010; Gibbs 2001; Probyn 2005). Gorton explains: 'As Williams points out, these texts' ability to "jerk" emotion from us lead to their cultural devaluation and to the perception that they are not "good" for us, and, I would argue, a sense that we should feel ashamed or even angry if they have managed to make us cry or scream' (in Gorton 2009, 79). Many of the participants regarded *The New Normal* as an inferior media artefact, which reflected a similar response to reality TV show *Giuliana & Bill* as discussed in the previous chapter. It was described as 'crap… I didn't like the way they developed the characters, the dialogue, the way it was filmed' (Laura, non-mothers focus group), and 'cheesy… I didn't like the way the cameras were zooming around' (Rose, pre-mothers focus group). Although *The New Normal* attempted to integrate the more realist cinema verité style of observational documentary through the 'zooming around' of what meant to appear as hand-held cameras, a common feature of reality TV, the result was not convincing. Instead of emotionally engaging with viewers, many of the participants disengaged.

However, through the evocation of the shock emotion, and through the genre technique of anxious displacements, Bryan and David's queerness is eradicated, minimised. I argue this legitimises gay parenting, which positions them as good, acceptable homosexuals. I propose this method of eradication resonates with what I have named a *queer straightness*. Despite homosexuality being normalised by positioning the characters in proximity to signs of straightness/happiness—such as family and children—and the anxiety of difference is displaced onto the surrounding characters, these representations are still problematic as they are both progressive and regressive, which I propose reinforces negative images of homosexuality. Carrie (mixed mothers focus group) believed that 'dealing with a gay couple makes it more palatable for the audience'. Here she is describing that the practice of surrogacy is more easily understood as a more viable option due to two men's reproductive restrictions. Furthermore, what can also be identified in her comment is that for homosexuals to be positioned as central characters on a prime-time TV show, particularly as soon-to-be parents, being in a couple makes *both* homosexuality and gay parenting more acceptable, and less deviant, for mainstream audiences.

The couple dyad is central to both the love plot, and normative personhood. What is of interest here in the context of *The New Normal* is how the coupling of homosexual men in relation to creating a family with a genetic bond, makes them, as Carrie observed, more palatable. I argue the couple configuration has drawn on the mother/father dualism that is central to the sitcom formula. I believe that the emergence of this dualism within the articulation of same-sex relationships encapsulates traditional notions of femininity and masculinity, in relation to parental roles within the family home. This I explore through elements of the butch–femme model, which although it belongs to lesbian culture, has explanatory value here. This model has been used to describe gay male masculinity, but the use of butch–femme to describe the dynamic of homosexual relationships has not been used to same extent (Ward 2008).

Sally R. Munt (1998) has described butch–femme as having gender characteristics that express one's identity through the performative—creating ways to look, and be looked at, as a conceptual way of speaking.

The butch–femme binary is complex, and has been a contentious category within lesbian culture, primarily critiqued by lesbian feminists in the 1970s–1980s for aping heterosexuality (Halberstam 1998; Munt 1998, 2008). I argue that traces of this model appear in the construction of the homosexual couple, which I propose produces, or speaks, an acceptable mode of homosexual parenting by drawing on the gender stereotyping of mother/father roles.

This, I also believe, in support of the butch–femme critique, also mimics hetero-norms. This resonates with Alexander Doty's (2010) reading of the homosexual couple in *Modern Family*, whom he asserts are characters shaped as '"good gays" able to keep their "place at the table" by striving to be just like their straight middle class counterparts, living in a monogamous relationship and building up a (mildly dysfunctional) family with children, a stay-at-home "mom," and a working "dad"' (in Pugh 2018, 176). As has been argued, these are antiquated gender roles that have been reinstated to make gay parenting more acceptable (LaVecchia 2011; Pugh 2018).

David is fit, masculine, successful and good-looking, which I argue positions him as the butch in the pairing. Fred Fejes (2000) claims that by constructing gay male characters in this way makes them more accessible to mainstream heterosexual audiences. Fejes claims this is done by portraying homosexual men as 'young, white, Caucasian, preferably with a well muscled, smooth body, handsome face, good education, professional job, and a high income' (2000, 15). As stated earlier in the chapter, the emergence of homosexual couples as parents has only recently become visible on prime-time television and film, which further shapes them as ideal, normal types of homosexuals. Guillermo Avila-Saavedra (2009) argues in his discussion of the increasing visibility of homosexual characters in the American popular media: 'Homosexual images are presented in a way acceptable for heterosexual audiences by reinforcing traditional values like family, monogamy and stability. Most of the erotic connotations of homosexuality have been eliminated' (2009, 8). This erasure of homosexual eroticism is discussed towards the end of the chapter.

As well as being shaped as the more masculine of the couple, David is also characterised as possessing fewer gay traits than his partner, Bryan. David's only friends are the straight men he works with. Bryan teases him relentlessly for his lack of popular cultural gay knowledge, and in the flashback scene which showed how the pair first met, in a gay bar,

David appears 'straight' and out of place. In contrast, Bryan's character is constructed as more effeminate, although not depicted as the 'swishy effeminate queen' (Walters 2001, 61) character that frequently appears in sitcoms. Homosexuality and effeminacy, much like lesbianism and masculinity, is a trait that has been integral to gay male stereotyping since the 1960s, when homosexual characters first appeared on TV (Dyer 1977, 2012; Gross and Woods 1999). This stereotyping is still prevalent, identified in fairly recent hit shows like *Will & Grace* where the majority of the gay characters were overly feminised (Linneman 2008). It can be argued that such stereotyping is rooted in late nineteenth and early twentieth-century models of gender inversion, where it was believed that gender traits in homosexuals and lesbians were reversed (Martin 1997; Sedgwick 2008).

Bryan's character is positioned in the feminine role, as the femme, through conventional articulations of normative feminine ideals, such as the disciplinary practice of dieting, the desire for family and marriage, and an unquenchable thirst for shopping (Bartky 1991; Dowling 2003; Friedan 2010). It is conceivable to suggest that this compliance to gender norms demonstrates what is required to be deemed a good mother (Feasey 2013).

In one scene, Bryan (although David also tries it on) is shown sporting a 'milk man'—a vest with built-in nipples (Season 1, Episode 15: 'Dairy Queen'). This version of femininity can be viewed as an imitation of heterosexual femininity, which situates a non-masculine gayness in the shadow of heterosexuality (Battles and Hilton-Morrow 2002; Butler 1993). Through this femme positioning, in the reflection of David's butch persona, the pair also mirror a similar butch–femme dynamic that is evident in the portrayal of Mitch and Cam in *Modern Family*. Mitch performs the more masculine role by being a successful lawyer in a hetero-dominant space, and Cam is a music teacher who stays at home to look after their adopted baby. Peter Kunze (2013) claims that the writers of *Modern Family* constructed the dynamic between the two men in the reflection of the heterosexual couples, 'so that the heterosexual norm is reinforced and idolized' (in Demory and Pullen 2013, 108). Like Bryan, I argue that Cam's character is positioned as the 'femme' through the display of overly camp character traits, and how he has been situated as the primary caregiver within the family home. This is also an example of how television continues to cultivate such gendered assumptions, regardless of how 'modern' the shows appear to be, primarily through the core ideas that 'women are happiest at home raising children' and 'men are born with more ambition than women' (Morgan 1982 in Feasey 2013, 186).

However, it is Bryan's positioning as the mother, the femme, in the relationship with David, the butch, which is troubling. Although there has been a strong argument made in lesbian culture that butch–femme is subversive, not mimicking but highlighting the excess of heterosexuality for erotic sexual play/desire (Butler 1990; De Lauretis 1994; Roof 1998), I believe that Bryan's femme character is assimilating into the heterosexual model rather than subverting it. As Judith Butler (1990) argues, butch–femme aims to destabilise identities, not conform to heterosexual terms. I argue that the materialisation of butch–femme within the characters of David and Bryan is doing the opposite.

The character constructions in *The New Normal* not only perpetuate an acceptable homosexuality but also, due to being situated within the mother/father sitcom binary, are misogynistic, as they also reinforce normative ideals of femininity and gender roles within discourses of family. Furthermore, through anxious displacements and the use of the stereotype, the surrounding characters are positioned as deviant, particularly working-class women (Goldie) and women of colour (Rocky).

Crying Like a Girl

> She turned more into a woman, into a straight woman. She turned more girly. That's what she said.
>
> (Rachel, non-mothers focus group, 2015)

The focus of this section is to explore the representation of the lesbian identified character Brenda[3] in *Rules of Engagement*. A key storyline that emerges in seasons 5–7 is that after several years struggling with infertility, lead character Audrey and her husband Jeff search for a surrogate to carry their genetic child. Jeff's best friend Brenda volunteers her services. During the early stages of pregnancy, Brenda struggles with sickness, and splits from her partner. The couple move Brenda into their home until the baby is delivered. Brenda agrees to be their surrogate in the episode entitled 'Les-Bro' (Season 5, Episode 8), a title that has clearly been derived from the homophobic lesbian slang 'lesbo'. This title portrays Brenda as a masculine woman, a common stereotype used to identify members of lesbian subculture.

Like Bryan in *The New Normal*, whose femme persona was constructed by drawing on normative feminine traits, Brenda's character is drawn from cultural stereotypes that are core to normative masculinity. Her character dresses in jeans, plaid shirts, and the laughter track chuckles on queue when she tells Audrey she shops at Bloomingdale's men's shoe department. As Tara (non-mothers focus group) surmised from reading Brenda's character: 'Apparently, as a lesbian you don't have any woman traits, which was very stereotypical'.

Although it has been argued that the sitcom convention of the stereotype is used to lampoon members of minority groups, and acts as a tool to uphold dominant ideological norms (Mills 2005, 2009), it has also been proposed—particularly in relation to gay stereotyping on TV (Dyer 1993)—that humour is a way to publicly expose and explore difficult subjects, which in this context can include reproductive practices such as surrogacy. As previously emphasised, sitcoms often employ stereotypes of the effeminate male and the butch female to make fun of lesbians and gay men, which preserves negative stereotypes. However, as Carla (mixed mothers focus group) pinpoints, lesbian characters are more prone to ridicule: 'Everyone can still laugh at lesbians, right? It's the thing on telly'. This illustrates how lesbian sexuality is played for laughs on mainstream television (Moritz 1987, 1999). Furthermore, this also demonstrates how humour can—but not always, depending on the text and the context (Douglas 1968)—be exposed as far from trivial by its ability to shape identities, social relationships and social interaction (Lockyer and Pickering 2008).

Like Jeff, Brenda likes drinking beer and watching sports, frequent activities the pair share which binds their friendship, leading up to the pregnancy. Their friendship sparked when they met on their local softball team. As identified by Rebecca Feasey (2008) in her work on masculinity and television advertising, but which can be applied here, drinking beer is positioned as core to normative masculinity by representing camaraderie. Jeff is a classic representative of dominant notions of masculinity by being constructed as the 'jock'—white, heterosexual, with a naturalised supremacy over women. He assumes a hierarchical position through the subordination of others, by gay baiting and making misogynistic comments (Charlebois 2011; Connell and Messerschmidt 2005).

Throughout the show, Jeff makes comments about Brenda such as 'she's not my wife, she's a lesbian' (Season 7, Episode 13: '100th'), and 'we have a mutual fondness for a nice rack' (Season 5, Episode 14:

'Uh-oh It's Magic'). These statements exclude her from the category 'woman' by positioning her as masculine. However, although Brenda's character is derived from stereotypes of normative masculinity, her character has not been portrayed through the commonly adopted trope of the butch lesbian. Although Brenda's character is shaped through mannish traits, she wears make-up and has long groomed hair, which are the conventional markings of normative femininity—codes that must be adhered to by lesbian characters to feature on prime-time TV and to avoid audience alienation (Lewis and Scanlon 2016; Moritz 1987, 1999). Drawing on the work of Susan J. Wolfe and Lee Ann Roripaugh (2006) and Martin Zeller-Jacques (2011), I propose that Brenda is performing within what the programmes have constructed to be a post-lesbian environment, where 'a certain type of lesbian is accepted' (Zeller-Jacques 2011, 104).

In contrast, the butch lesbian is constructed with a more muscular or larger frame, short hair and no make-up. This is a stereotypical image which Judith Halberstam (1998) describes as 'identity in excess', which she argues is troublesome as it makes, 'lesbianism readable in the register of masculinity' (2008, 177). This correlates with the notion that lesbians are not, and cannot be, feminine, as they are unable to have 'any woman traits' (Tara, non-mothers focus group). During the viewing session of *The New Normal*, Carrie (heterosexual) and Jackie (bisexual) (mixed mothers focus group) were both irritated by a scene that showed the surrogate's grandmother 'Nana' was revolted by seeing a butch lesbian couple who she described as 'ugly men' strolling in public with their baby (Episode 1: 'Pilot').

> Carrie: Yeah, that's right, that's how lesbians are *always* portrayed.
> Jackie: That's a lesbian couple? Right… of course, the butch lesbian couple.
> (Carrie and Jackie, mixed mothers focus group, 2015)

Jackie, who identifies as bisexual, was particularly perturbed by the butch lesbian representation. She stated how much it annoyed her 'how lesbians were always stereotyped' in this way. Richard Dyer (1977) claims in his work on the representation of gays in film that such stereotypes *do* exist within subcultures and are therefore representatives of these minority groups. Yet, despite Brenda's masculine traits, which are still problematic as they are built on the stereotype of lesbian masculinity, it could be argued that her character is challenging the image of the butch lesbian, by being constructed as what Halberstam (1998) describes as a 'barely butch'—a representation of the everyday lesbian who may not appear conventionally butch, but 'might do something considered to be traditionally male' (1998, 217–218). In Brenda's case, this is drinking beer and watching sports.

However, in relation to the surrogacy storyline, what *is* revealing is how Brenda, as a barely butch, is assimilated into heterosexual culture, by being taken into the heterosexual couple's home—the heterosexual couple being the central point where 'the world unfolds' (Ahmed 2006, 85). Brenda is integrated into their friendship circle, as what appears to be the token gay person.[4] This she disrupts through pregnancy, which in addition disturbs the lesbian subject position through the social and cultural assumptions that pregnancy and motherhood are located within the heterosexual domain (Calhoun 2000). Brenda is not positioned on the outside, as the deviant butch lesbian, a character often situated in prison (*Prisoner: Cell Block H, Bad Girls, Caged! Orange Is the New Black*), but on the inside of dominant heterosexual culture.

For a lesbian to be assimilated into dominant heterosexual culture is only made possible not only by reducing signs of gayness (Moritz 1987, 1999) but also by erasing any references to a vibrant gay community which the characters may be a part of. This is also seen in *The New Normal*. I propose this absence supports heterosexual dominance (Cavalcante 2014; Walters 2001, 2012). However, the butch lesbian is positioned as non-normative by failing to assimilate, often rendered invisible through death, misconduct, shame or scandal (Halberstam 1998; Kuhn 1992; Moritz 1987, 1999).

Brenda's character is portrayed as more acceptable through not only the barely butch image of the everyday lesbian but also through her ability to get pregnant, which, drawing Ellen Lewin's (1993) work on lesbian motherhood, makes her lesbianism more tolerable by straight communities. In this representation, however, pregnancy is temporary—Brenda has no desire to be a mother, to be discussed below. Brenda's character could be viewed as a form of progression in representation on one hand, by breaking down homophobic stereotyping of lesbianism and making visible more varied lesbian identities. Or, it could be viewed as erasing what has been argued as actual representations of a type of lesbian masculinity (Dyer 1977; Halberstam 1998) in favour of a version that is more agreeable for mainstream audiences, also seen in the characters of Will in *Will and Grace*, and David in *The New Normal*.

Brenda is portrayed in *Rules of Engagement* similarly to the lesbian characters in *The L Word*. It has been argued that the *L Word* lacks a range of diversity by the characters being white, middle class and femme (Lewis and Scanlon 2016), and positioned within heterosexual narratives such as domesticity, romance and reproduction, for heterosexual audiences (Wolfe and Roripaugh in Akass and McCabe 2006; Lee and Meyer 2010). However, as pointed out by Ron Becker (2006) in his work on gay television in straight America, some mainstream networks and their advertisers were keen to target a very specific gay audience, one that is white, affluent and well educated which does not reflect the diversity of gay communities. As Becker argues: 'gay material was used to target a significantly larger audience of socially liberal, urban-minded professionals' (2006, 177).

In relation to gay articulations in mainstream culture, Amy Villarejo (2003) highlights in her analysis of lesbian images in film how lesbian chic has 'crept into national culture and commodity culture' (2003, 7); a new visibility that has emerged to help sell cultural products such as film, books, photography and video. However, as proposed by Wolfe and Roripaugh (2006) in their analysis of the *L Word*, this type of visibility has caused anxiety amid lesbian viewers, through a pandering to the heterosexual gaze, the result of which they claim are inauthentic depictions of lesbian identities. As lesbian journalist Winnie McCroy expressed in her review of the *L Word* in LGBTQ newspaper *The New York Blade* (2004):

> If lesbians have to choose between remaining invisible to the mainstream, or being represented by Showtime's clipped and plucked lesbians, I choose invisibility. After all, real lesbians will still remain invisible, at least until our lives become more than a marketing tool or cottage industry or pud fodder for Joe Sixpack. (in Akass and McCabe 2006, 44)

Brenda in *Rules of Engagement* is a *visible* mainstream lesbian, a barely butch character positioned within a central narrative of family and reproduction, that is *just* feminine enough for audiences to read as a woman with a viable uterus (which defines womanhood). However, Brenda's characteristics are also masculine enough to not create anxieties in relation to the ethics of surrogacy, and any potential claims on the baby. I argue, therefore, that the representation of Brenda in relation to motherhood draws on the social and cultural notions that view the lesbian as not a *real* woman, which, alongside lesbianism and motherhood, is discussed further in Chapter 4. I propose that through this depiction of lesbianism the mother–child bond is eradicated—Brenda is not depicted as a *real* mother, either. As Rebecca (non-mothers focus group) commented:

> People just assume that normal people wouldn't necessarily want to say… "OK you can borrow my womb for a bit and I'll have a baby for you". It has to be for some other reason.
>
> (Rebecca, non-mothers focus group, 2015)

I propose that this 'other reason' Rebecca is describing is the lesbian body, which is positioned as non-normative by associating 'normal people' with normative heterosexuality. This further suggests that the lesbian is not considered a real woman, positioned outside of the category 'woman', and is therefore able to loan her body as a container. Through this commentary, the resistors' (Lam 2015) feminist critique of reproductive technologies can be evoked, where it was argued that women's bodies were thought of as holding vessels, foetal containers—maternal subjectivity made invisible. As the only lesbian surrogate depicted in the material under analysis, Brenda appears the most emotionally unattached to, and disinterested in, the baby she carried and delivered, with no interest in being a mother, either. This articulation resonates with the notion that lesbian mothers are seen as unfit mothers—women who are monsters and freaks who threaten the structures of heteronormative culture (Allison 1996; Sourbut 1996; Throsby 2004). Despite, in reality, the number of lesbian mothers being on the increase, they are still rarely shown on television as are considered improper for family audiences (Feasey 2015; Kinnick 2009).

The changes of Brenda's character traits through the experience of pregnancy were of particular interest to the focus group participants, especially one scene (Season 5, Episode 20: 'Beating the System'), where Brenda, newly pregnant, meets Jeff in the local diner. She has an emotional meltdown after a bout of morning sickness. In tears, she turns to Jeff and sobs: 'Thanks a lot Jeff, you've turned me into a frickin' girl!' As the 'jock' Jeff is presented as being emotionally distanced—he struggles to show empathy. As soon as Brenda leaves the diner, he turns to his friends and says: 'I've never seen her so unreasonable and cranky, she's being really wifey'. Carrie, Carla and Sonja (mixed mothers focus group) chose to discuss this scene in relation to sexuality, pregnancy and femininity:

> Carrie: For me, I think the lesbian surrogate is really interesting as it's this idea that the pregnancy hormones made her somehow feminine.
> Sonja: Yeah, yeah, yeah…
> Carla: But that meant being mental, and emotional -- a pain in the arse.
> Sonja: Yeah, and crying… because, if you're a gay woman then you're as hard as nails, and you're not going to cry.
> Carrie: You're not really a woman.
> (Carrie, Carla and Sonja, mixed mothers focus group, 2015)

These comments resonate with Halberstam's (1998) argument that lesbianism cannot be read as anything other than masculine in mainstream culture, which draws on conventional notions of masculinity (Sonja: 'if you're a gay woman you're as hard as nails, and you're not going to cry'). Furthermore, what can also be recognised is how the experience of pregnancy, as a heterosexual narrative—as also seen in *The L Word*—performs as a straightening device, which develops from Ahmed's (2010) argument that being in the proximity of signs of straightness (in this context, pregnancy, family) minimises signs of homosexuality/lesbianism. The pregnancy hormones have, as Carrie stated: 'made her somehow feminine' (which reads as straight). Pregnancy has removed Brenda from the non-normative, deviant position of the lesbian—who's not a *real* woman—and has repositioned her as nearly normative, or as described by Kate McNicholas Smith and Imogen Tyler (2017) the 'lesbian normal'. The lesbian normal, in their explanation, is a carefully crafted popular cultural articulation of modern feminine lesbianism, made acceptable for mainstream audiences, 'which affirm ideals of hetero-patriarchal, white, middle-class femininity' (2017, 3). Brenda is positioned on the right path paved by compulsory heterosexuality, a default patriarchal structure that disciplines women's sexuality to channel them into the institutions of motherhood and marriage (Ahmed 2006; Rich 1980).

Although Brenda is not the genetic mother, and is not to be the child's caretaker, Rich's (1980) argument that motherhood, like heterosexuality, is a political institution is worth considering. Rich proposes that the two are inextricably linked through what she argues is a societal force that traditionally privileges male power over women. Rich also claims that through this force, lesbianism becomes obscured. Brenda's lesbianism is made more invisible, albeit temporarily. Although she does not become romantically partnered during this period—her lesbian desire is blocked, which will be discussed in the next section—she is taken into the heterosexual couple's home when she becomes pregnant. I argue this socialises her into the heteronormative sphere, which again positions her in proximity to signs of straightness, to kinship objects that as Ahmed (2006) argues, *do* the work of family. As Jeff pinpoints after Brenda's emotional outburst in the diner, she has transitioned from his drinking buddy to being 'really wifey'.

Symbolically, there is a scene (Season 5, Episode 20: 'Beating the System') where Audrey discovers Jeff is not running errands, but has, instead, retreated to his office to escape Brenda's mood swings. Audrey admits she too is struggling with Brenda's emotional outbursts. The pair therefore hide out in the office. This suggests that Brenda, through her new feminine identity, has shifted to the wife, and the wife has shifted to the buddy, which indicates that Audrey has been situated in a more masculine position, like the father, as she is removed from the gestational role. This notion of the paternal positioning of women is discussed further in the following chapter. Pregnancy, therefore, has made Brenda a *real* woman, which has been proposed is the basis of being female (Brook 1999). It can be argued, then, that this transformation conforms to normative notions of hetero-femininity, through the excess of emotions that have surfaced through pregnancy. These emotional characteristics have traditionally been associated with normative notions of 'womanhood', specifically in relation to heterosexual women (in Martin 1997): lesbians, like men, being 'as hard as nails'. Women have also been historically linked to what has been constructed as a natural femininity, rather than cultural masculinity, as informed by the Cartesian binary of nature/culture, which positions normative femininity with the naturalness of reproduction.

Brenda's character highlights this gender construct through transitioning from masculine to feminine, non-woman to real woman, rational to irrational. Not only does this construction depict femininity as weak under conventional notions of femininity, which is demonstrated in this text, but it also points to what has been described by feminist scholars as an unsettling experience of pregnancy, where the female body is split, doubled, and the female subject is no longer experiencing herself, as herself (Kristeva 1980; Young 1984). In this context, Brenda no longer feels like a lesbian, she feels straight. This counters Ahmed's proposition that happiness causes, such as 'the family, marriage, whiteness' (2010, 112), promise happiness to the deviant queer. This appears as not the case in this representation—Brenda's proximity to social norms have, in fact, made her unhappy. She dislikes the changes in her emotions, she dislikes not being able to drink beer, she dislikes feeling more feminine and she wants the baby out of her body and into Audrey's arms, as soon as possible. This accentuates the heterosexist belief that lesbians are not fit to be mothers, viewed as socially and culturally incompatible with motherhood. The lesbian can't be shown as *wanting* to be a mother as motherhood is a natural, normative desire, which the lesbian, who is positioned as non-normative, should be excluded from, due to being viewed as inferior.

In addition, it can also be proposed that the experience of pregnancy, which is symbolic of conventional heterosexual ritual, has transported Brenda's lesbian body into what could be described, drawing on Michel Foucault (1984) and José Muñoz (2009) as what I call heterotopic straight time. According to Foucault, the heterotopic space is an in-between space, such as the prison, which he argued is a parallel space (also a ship, asylum) which requires a form of membership. Foucault argued that these places are constructed to control undesirable bodies, which therefore makes the concept of utopia possible. For the purpose of this discussion, I argue that the lesbian is the deviant body, and utopia is a dominant heterosexual culture. Within this framework I argue that through the experience of pregnancy, the deviant body of the lesbian enters the straight time (Muñoz) of heterosexual reproduction—pregnancy representative of a heterotopic space (Foucault), the straight time being the temporal heterosexual sphere that Brenda enters.

Muñoz proposes that the queer is already in straight time and wishes to step out of it, into a queer futurity. I suggest in this analysis that the queer—in this context, the lesbian—steps into the straight time of pregnancy. I propose that the body of the deviant lesbian (heterotopic space) is a vehicle by which to produce future subjects for a future world (utopia). Through her desire to be a surrogate, Brenda has not been able to resist straight time's pull into heterosexual reproduction, which could be read as a desire for validation, to be recognised as a good homosexual (Ahmed 2010; Seidman 2004). This resonates with Ahmed's argument of how one dwells in one's body, and how one inhabits spaces, can act as an orientation device (Ahmed 2006). Therefore, this transition through pregnancy, regardless of the lesbian surrogate not carrying her own genetic foetus, can also be read as men's power over women, through the impregnation of his seed (the future)—the female body being the material component (the space), the male seed providing the creative power, giving it life and force (Colebrook 2003).

Rachel (non-mothers focus group), who is lesbian-identified, read the scene that indicated the shift in Brenda's character traits from masculine to feminine through pregnancy, differently:

> This shows the typical male ideal about how a lesbian woman just needs a good seeing to by a man, and she'll become feminine, and not liking dick, basically – that's what this means.
>
> (Rachel, non-mothers focus group, 2015)

Although it appears that Rachel has misunderstood that the surrogacy arrangement in this narrative is executed through the non-coital method of embryo transfer, and not the natural method of sexual intercourse, she is signalling towards the radical lesbian feminist perspective that the true essence of being a 'woman' is to be penetrated by men (Radicalesbians 1970).

Furthermore, through her comment, the common popular cultural and societal belief that lesbianism is just a temporary phase can also be identified. This frequently emerges in and is constructed by media representations, inferring that lesbianism is due to either the lack of men, or not being able to 'get' a man (Ahmed 2006; Freud 1977). As Rachel highlighted, it is through the carrying of the male seed that Brenda will 'become feminine' (again, read as straight), which realigns the female body into the normative dimension of heterosexuality (Ahmed 2006). However, despite Rachel's reading—similarly to the lesbian being portrayed as happy, rather than unhappy—it transpires that in this character portrayal, it is heterosexuality, and not lesbianism, which is the temporary phase. The first thing Brenda says after the baby was born was: 'Thank God, I can drink again!' (Season 7, Episode 13: '100th'). This symbolises a return to her former masculine femininity, and a return to happiness. This was the final scene that featured Brenda. From this moment on, she was erased—once her services were completed. Not killed off, dishonoured or sent to prison, or as Ahmed also outlines, 'turn straight, die, or go mad' (Ahmed 2010, 89), but excluded from heteronormative membership, which is a common lesbian narrative in popular culture (Dyer 1977; Kaplan 1998; Stacey 1993).[5]

In the very final scene of the final episode of the show, the characters are pictured together, happily sharing the news that Audrey has fallen pregnant naturally, despite being told she was infertile. During Brenda's labour, Audrey discovers she is pregnant. This final equilibrium in the narrative suggests that the desired outcome is natural pregnancy through heterosexual sex, with the lesbian out of sight. Although Brenda's heteronormative membership was temporary, so was the lesbian visibility on a prime-time TV show, which was only enabled through the device of pregnancy as a normative journey, and as the central plot device built within a heterosexual narrative (Oliver 2012). Brenda's role was to enable a 'happy heterosexuality' (Ahmed 2010, 90) through her own sacrifice and by being inserted into the storyline as a sidekick, which is often deemed the most fitting role for gay characters (Schulman 1998). As Patricia White (1999) states in her work on lesbian representation in Hollywood cinema, the lesbian character has shifted from being the uninvited guest to being invited. But in the end, in *Rules of Engagement*, the invited guest was uninvited once more and shown the door.[6]

Fitting In

> It's not a gay or straight thing – the concept of family not being a family unless there are children involved.
>
> (Sonja, mixed mothers focus group, 2015)

In this statement, it can be suggested that Sonja is inferring that to be viewed as a proper, normative family, children must be included in the family frame. She has identified a societal and cultural shift, through the reading of *The New Normal* and *Rules of Engagement*, that the aspiration of the family ideal is not either gay or straight specific, but is pertinent to all, whether it be the homosexual couple in *The New Normal*, or the heterosexual couple in *Rules of Engagement*. As Sonja states, it is no longer a 'gay or straight thing'. Sonja's reading of the portrayal of both sets of couples supports the notion that in order for a family to be complete, it is necessary that the couple have children, otherwise they are not considered a *real* family (Benkov 1994; Burke 1993; Lehr 1999; Nelson 2007, 2009). Furthermore, Sonja's interpretation also suggests a belief that the child is the lynchpin of reproductive futurism—without the baby being central to the family unit, there is *no future*, no community, no national sanctity (Berlant 1994; Berlant and Warner 1998; Edelman 2003; Muñoz 2009).

However, what Lee Edelman (2003) has posed, is that despite the dominant belief that reproduction is associated with heterosexuality, members of the LGBTQ community are not exempt from being able to resist its appeal. As Muñoz (2007) argues, and which is useful to evoke here, there is a pull into what he calls straight time—as mentioned above—which is the here and now of everyday life, shaped by heterosexual reproduction. It is possible to suggest that this reflects, in part, the desire to be hetero-ordinary that far right gay commentators such as Andrew Sullivan (1995) have ardently fought for, proposing that some homosexuals *want* to avoid signs of gayness, and wish to be seen as ordinary—to be seen as straight(er). For Sullivan, to be ordinary is an aspiration, an accomplishment, to escape deviancy, isolation, and shame. He believes this has allowed him to integrate into mainstream society:

> Once I found the strength to be myself, I had no need to act myself. And it came as no surprise that once I had become more open about my homosexuality, these mannerisms declined. So my clothes became progressively more regular and slovenly; I lost interest in drama; my writing moved from fiction to journalism; my speech actually became less affected. (in Lehr 1999, 9)

To be ordinary in these terms means to become part of a respectable community, resulting in meaningful social cohesion (Ahmed 2006; Berlant and Warner 1998; Sullivan 1995; Warner 1999). This desire to assimilate into the mainstream—in this discussion, through the creation of family—is demonstrated in a conversation between Carla, Carrie and Jackie (mixed mothers focus group):

> Carla: It's a societal thing… Having kids is hard fucking work – everyone says that. There's this sort of buying into the ideal, that means you fit in some way, and that now includes gay men, lesbian women.
> Carrie: And it normalises gay people.
> Jackie: Because it makes them more acceptable.
> (Carla, Carrie and Jackie, mixed mothers focus group, 2015)

Not only have these women recognised in these texts that the social and cultural value of the family with children is a socially constructed ideal, which requires 'buying into', they have also described that it is only by following the heterosexual narrative that homosexuals and lesbians are able to 'fit', and become accepted, into normative culture.

This process of normalisation includes mimicking the conventional family structure (which can also be viewed as challenging it, to be discussed further on) through monogamy, the sentimentality of the couple dyad and the stability of the family home (Avila-Saavedra 2009). Therefore, it can be suggested that those who do not assimilate/conform to such a narrative are positioned as deviant, moored at the margins of normative culture, viewed as unnatural, bad citizens (Ahmed 2010; Rubin 2011; Seidman 2004; Warner 1999).

As has been discussed throughout this chapter, I propose that the narrative and characterisation in *The New Normal* and *Rules of Engagement* have been assembled to present a respectable version of homosexuality, enabled through an allegiance to the family ideal. What emerges is what I have named a *queer straightness*, which is where the characters' homosexual and lesbian traits and identities are normalised, straightened, which aims to soothe anxieties surrounding social differences by creating gay characters that are less threatening to mainstream culture. I argue this has been implemented primarily through the romance narrative, which shapes normative discourses of family and civilises sexual desire (Berlant 2011; Berlant and Warner 1998; Evans 2003).

By doing so, this also disciplines, or blocks, non-normative sexual practices by erasing same-sex intimacy through representation. In the context of the popular cultural articulations of homosexuality and lesbianism in this discussion, this emerges in *The New Normal* and *Rules of Engagement* by positioning the gay characters as parents—or in Brenda's case, pregnant–on prime-time TV. While these representations may appear progressive, I propose they are also regressive, as hetero-centricity drives the narrative structure and characterisation. David and Bryan in *The New Normal*, and Brenda in *Rules of Engagement* are positioned as acceptable *only* if sexual intimacy is made less visible than their heterosexual counterparts. Although the focus group participants didn't specifically pinpoint this division in relation to sexual intimacy, some described clear differences in how the characters were presented in relation to reproduction. Tara (non-mothers focus group) made a poignant observation:

> I think if I was a gay man and I was in that position I'd be a bit pissed off about that. It trivialised it [surrogacy] and made it, not... trying to divorce

> what heterosexuals' relationship are with children and what gay couples' relationships are with children.
>
> (Tara, non-mothers focus group, 2015)

Tara's comment implies a separate treatment of the heterosexual and homosexual characters' relationship to the building of the conventional construct of family. This can be developed further by identifying what I propose is a separate treatment of same-sex sexual intimacy on screen, which insinuates what *is* and *isn't* acceptable for mainstream viewing (and therefore, mainstream culture). For gay intimacy to be included on and seen as acceptable for prime-time television, for heterosexual audiences, it must be presented as less passionate and less sexual than normative heterosexuals (Bruni 1994; Moritz 1987, 1999; Rubin 2011), to the point where it is non-existent—if it is to be represented at all. Drawing on Eve Kosofsky Sedgwick (2008), this articulation of gay identity performs as a form of closeting, through silencing—an act of power which is rooted in the stigma of intimate same-sex relations.

In *Rules of Engagement*, Brenda's lesbian identity and sexual practices are submerged, or blocked, through the surrogate pregnancy that caused the break up with her sexual partner—normative heterosexual rituals, such as pregnancy, stopping sexual deviancy. Drawing on Marguerite J. Moritz (1999) analysis of lesbian representations on American TV drama *Hotel* (1983–1988), it can be suggested that this separation of Brenda from her lover performs as a term of acceptance for a lesbian character to be represented culturally—not through the death of the sexual partner, as Moritz describes in *Hotel,* but the death of the sexual relationship as the result of heterosexual dominance. This can be identified through the surveillance and control of Brenda's body, not only through the insemination process but also throughout the period Brenda is taken into the intended parents' home. It can be argued that this demonstrates a disciplinary power through the exertion of a dominant heterosexual power over an LGBTQ body. Drawing on Foucault (1977), the surrogate's body can be described as a docile body, a body that 'may be subjected, used, transformed and improved' (1977, 136). This is illustrated through the constant surveillance of Brenda's body, to optimise the body's capacities, to make it productive—to produce a child to enable a happy heterosexuality.[7] The heterosexual couple's family is completed (normalised) while the lesbian surrogate remains uncoupled, and a non-mother (deviant).

Similarly, Bryan and David in *The New Normal* invite their surrogate, Goldie, into their home during the term of her pregnancy. They swap her fast food diet for organic food, which implies class differences, to be discussed in the following chapter. They too are exerting dominant heteronormativity over their surrogate, as they are adhering to the sameness of heterosexual norms. This reflects Lisa Duggan's concept of *homonormativity*, which is 'a politics that does not contest dominant heteronormative assumptions and institutions, but upholds and sustains them, while promising the possibility of a demobilized gay constituency and a privatized, depoliticized gay culture anchored in domesticity and consumption' (Duggan 2002, 50).

Although the surrogate, Goldie, in *The New Normal* is heterosexual, it can be argued that she is also positioned as deviant due to her being an uneducated and unskilled single mother, who is not trusted to nourish the growing foetus and seen as incapable of parenting her young daughter. Goldie does not live up to the idealised maternal role, therefore as a docile body under the surveillance and intervention of two middle-class white gay men, she has the potential to improve. Drawing on Katherine Kinnick (2009), the narrative here 'casts motherhood in moral terms' (2009, 3) as Goldie is painted as a bad mother. Not only is she single, but she also lacks ambition, is of a lower-income status, and does not conform to traditional maternal behaviour.[8] Kinnick explains this is articulated through the juxtaposition of the good mother/bad mother. The good mother(s) in this TV text being the Bryan and David who step into show her how it's done. Like Brenda in *Rules of Engagement*, Goldie is also too enabling what I call a *happy homonormativity* for the homosexual men, by providing them a child.

Gay men make up just over half of the representations of LGBTQ characters on prime-time TV. Queer media scholars who have explored these representations have highlighted that relationships between men are reduced to moments of male bonding, a peck on the cheek, a passionless embrace (Aslinger 2013; Battles and Hilton-Morrow 2015; Moritz 1987, 1999; Lucas and Raley 2006). This dilution of sexual intimacy is most prevalent within the sitcom, due to the genre's stricter boundaries, which are set in place to attract, and seek approval from, what has been described as the mainstream heterosexual gaze (Cavalcante 2014; Dow 1996, 2001). As American TV columnist Gail Shister expressed about the lack of same-sex sexual intimacy shown on popular TV shows: 'Sure, it's OK to be gay; it may even be OK to have kids. But it's not OK to have sex' (in Frutkin 1995, 31). This reflects the homophobic notion that homosexual sexual acts should be kept in private, unseen, left to a shady existence (Foucault 1998; McKee 1996). It can be argued that this also illustrates what Foucault described as a shift in thought in the nineteenth century, that viewed homosexuality as an identity, rather than purely a sexual act—and what emerged was a newer category of person, a species, which formed the divisive binary of heterosexual/homosexual (Foucault 1998; Sedgwick 2008). This therefore signals that heterosexual sex is situated as the desired norm, erasing same-sex sexual presence, perpetuating a heteronormativity that asserts sameness to an idealised white, middle-class, heterosexual norm (Duggan 2002; Richardson 2005; Warner 1999). Heteronormativity saturates every aspect of the social and political sphere, from law and commerce to education and the media. This signifies what is deemed as correct behaviour, which is at the core of the institution of heterosexuality (Ahmed 2006; Berlant and Warner 1998; Rich 1980).

Although Rich's proposition of compulsory heterosexuality centred on men's power over women and the rendering invisible of the lesbian possibility, her proposal that the idealisation of heterosexuality acts as a societal force for social acceptance can be applied here. What has been identified in previous analyses of the gay male couples in both *The New Normal* and *Modern Family*, is that as gay parents they are only permitted to be like the straights as far as being positioned in a marriage-type relationship, as good neighbours, with social worth and economic status (Cavalcante 2014; Kunze 2013), which as Jackie (mixed mothers focus group) observed, 'makes them more acceptable'. These images of the 'normal' homosexuals portrayed in these texts typify the beliefs of the far-right gay movement that emerged in the United States post the Stonewall riots of 1969, and in the trail of homophile organisation the Mattachine Society, whose primary manifesto was that integration into dominant heterosexual society was key to achieve normative status.

This turning point in far-right gay activism was led by white, educated, economically mobile gay men whose desire for normativity was dependent on regarding sexuality and the sex act as irrelevant in the fight for equal rights (Warner 1999). This resonates with Duane Gilson's (2016) belief that 'queerness is not threatened most by heteronormativity, but by homonormativity, not by people outside of the LGBT community, but by the most powerful class, white gay men, inside of it' (2016, 24). In addition, this also echoes Foucault's observation of the shift from the genital sexual act to identity. However, sameness and equality are not evident here. The straight couples in *Modern Family* are often shown in intimate sexual situations, whereas the gay couple's intimacy was 'occluded from view' (Pugh 2018, 162). This de-sexualising of the couple caused some viewers disappointment—it took a Facebook campaign by the show's gay fans for the producers to include a kiss between the two men (Hilton-Morrow 2015; Pugh 2018). Even then, when it did happen, the kiss was a peck on the mouth.

Over two decades earlier, in 1989, hit American TV drama *Thirtysomething* (Season 3, Episode 6: 'Strangers') showed two men in bed together, after sex. As Frank Bruni (1994) recalls: 'Protests from viewers and sponsors made ABC pull the episode from syndication, never to be broadcast again' (1994, 328). As argued by Alan McKee (1996): 'Gay people have been visible as people, but not as gay. Homosexuality is proclaimed rather than performed; tongues are used to make passionate speeches, but not to deep-kiss gay lovers' (1996, 58).

This fear of showing intimacy between gay couples emerges in the narrative of *The New Normal*. David and Bryan's sexually intimate relations are regulated, despite the pair being situated within a monogamous relationship, with a desire for marriage and children—normal homosexuals who are 'the good and acceptable face of the movement' (Warner 1999, 66). However, how the kiss presents itself in various scenes throughout the series is symbolic of a new form of acceptable homosexuality, which has been situated within the heteronormative family framework. The kiss, as argued by McKee, is powerful because it is a signifier embedded with multiple connotations. In *The New Normal*, however, I argue the kiss signals a form of good homosexuality, one that is non-sexual and located within the narrative of family.

There are a number of key scenes that illustrate this. In the first bedroom scene, Bryan and David are dressed, sitting on their bed, picking out their egg donor and discussing who, out of the two of them, should provide the sperm. Soon after, they are pictured lying on the bed in an intimate embrace. They kiss, briefly (Season 1, Episode 1: 'Pilot'). The second kiss takes place in the nightclub where they first met, which they revisit in an attempt to capture their lost youth. The kiss arises during a nostalgic discussion of love, family and growing old together (Season 1, Episode 2: 'Sofa's Choice'). The third kiss appears in a baby clothes section at a shopping mall (Season 1, Episode 3: 'Baby Clothes'), and the fourth when David recounts the moment when he heard the baby's heartbeat for the first time: 'When we heard that heartbeat yesterday, I don't think I've ever loved you more' (Season 1, Episode 4: 'Obama Mama'). As McKee states: 'the kiss is a communicative act: it says something… it speaks to the people watching you kissing' (1996, 51).

In *The New Normal* the kiss is symbolic of romantic love, which is core to the heterosexual love plot, and which only emerges during sentimental scenes where the future child, embedded with hope and promise, is central. When David proposes to Bryan (Season 1, Episode 6: 'Bryanzilla'), he does so in front of the surrogate with a 3D ultrasound scan of the foetus in utero. David says to Bryan, while down on one knee, which mimics heterosexual ritual: 'I want our baby to be able to say: "I was there when my daddies got engaged"'. This scene illustrates how the technology of foetal imaging has created a visual culture of pregnancy that views the female body and foetus as conceptually separate, which, as has been argued, reduces the female body to a container, and positions the foetus as a subject, before birth. Moments before the proposal, the surrogate Goldie says: 'Just pretend I'm not here'. This further marks her as merely the container, which, as argued by a wide range of feminists, renders her invisible.

This kiss, therefore, is not only the signifier of true love, but is representative of an unthreatening and sentimental love that is deeply rooted in the narrative of family.[9] Berlant (2008) proposes that the sentimentality of the love plot is a project of femininity, which aims to centre women in the ideology of normative love. This she proposes is structured through the story of family and romance, which the woman must be emotionally invested in, as Carla (mixed mothers focus group) stated, 'buying into' the ideal, a fantasy that one must be invested into be happy, to be included, to be valued.

Extending Berlant's argument, it can be proposed that the romance narrative between the two gay men in *The New Normal*, in the context of building a family though surrogacy, is an example of how, as she says, popular culture has reinvented the love plot as a figure of optimism which is transformative. On the premise that one is wholly invested, normative love then has the power to 'rescue you from your life and give you a new one' (2008, 171). In *The New Normal,* normative love has been positioned as a central genre device, mobilised in ways that not only mould an acceptable version of homosexuality, but in doing so also rescues the homosexual from the shame of deviant sexual practice, promiscuity, non-procreation—and realigns them on the straight path through conforming to heteronormative ideals. These narratives reflect what Sarah Schulman (1998) calls a 'fake public homosexuality', one of its integral components being that 'gay content is only permissible if it focusses on romance' (1998, 147).

However, what has been identified, in the analysis of *The New Normal* in particular, is a shift from what has been described in shows such as *Will & Grace* as a twist on the delayed consummation plotline, which is where the interaction of characters is driven by sexual tension and the search for a romantic relationship. Where classical Hollywood narratives once centred on the male lead's desire to consummate the relationship and the female lead's desire to be wed, which was later adopted by the sitcom, the relationship between Will and Grace provided a new twist, separating possible lovers through sexual orientation (Battles and Hilton-Morrow 2015; Scodari 1995). I argue that this trope has been reinvented further, now replaced with what I call a delayed conception plotline, where the search for a sexual partner, or romantic love, has been replaced with the search for a child, through any means possible, even before the relationship is legitimated by marriage. In the final episode in *The New Normal* (Season 1, Episode 22: 'The Big Day'), the wedding between David and Bryan is played as a joke. As David says to a friend who showers him with confetti as he walks down the aisle: 'I'm pretty sure that's for after'. This both apes and mocks the heterosexual wedding ritual. However, the marriage is also blocked. Before the two men say, 'I do', Goldie's waters break which stops the marriage.

Despite challenging the nuclear family model through an attempt to destabilise heterosexual privilege through the construction of family built on not just same-sex parenting, but the alternative reproductive practice of surrogacy, the gay characters in *The New Normal* are not convincingly progressive. This is because they present a version of homosexuality that does not rupture the heteronormative fabric of mainstream society but does the work to maintain it. Even so, it must be acknowledged that the portrayal of Bryan and David are contributing to a new archive of images that McKee noted as absent two decades ago. In 1996, McKee believed that society found images of men kissing men on TV screens unthinkable, and even more unthinkable was that such kissing was able to signify 'the romance, the closeness, the dreams of relationships, which structure heterosexual television narrative' (1996, 70). As self-identified bisexual Jackie (mixed mothers focus group) stated, in response to the representations of homosexuality and lesbianism in both *The New Normal* and *Rules of Engagement*: 'I think it's better than not showing anything, I think things have come a long way, but it does still feel very stereotyped to me… this isn't real life for everybody'.

Jackie's sentiments express a desire to be seen on screen as a result of overwhelming invisibility (Pugh 2018) but also reflect the compromises made by 1950s fiction writer Vin Packer, who was forced to change the ending of her lesbian novel *Spring Fire* (1952) to enable 'a new book about us' (in Ahmed 2010, 89). What was originally a happy ending (women fall in love and stay together) became a miserable one (they break up due to mental illness). The publisher feared a happy ending would promote lesbianism. It seems remarkable that this 'better than nothing' response to media texts is still being expressed 65 years later.

Although heterosexual privilege has not been wholly challenged, and familial norms have been reproduced by adhering to the discourse of romantic love, at least these representations show advancement, with fewer portrayals of homosexual men as criminals, child molesters and predators (Lucas and Raley 2006; McKee 1996). However, this new representation of homosexuals and lesbians is still precarious.

As the research has revealed, to be acceptable, one has to be a certain type of gay man, situated within a monogamous couple dyad, adhering to conventional feminine/masculine gender roles—or, in the lesbian's case, a barely butch who is placed under surveillance for heterosexual reproduction. As highlighted by Dustin Bradley Goltz (2011), inclusionary practices, such as stretching heteronormativity to include gays, can also be exclusionary. I argue representations such as these exclude and make deviant any other forms of homosexuality, whose aspirations, or economic or racial status, do not permit them into the normative sphere—rent boys, drag queens, hookers, nelly boys, bulldaggers and welfare queens (Cohen 1997; Warner 1999). However, the category of heterosexuality must also be recognised in relation to being situated outside of dominant norms, as like homosexuality, heterosexuality is not monolithic. Heteronormative ideals can also alienate and make deviant heterosexuals who can't, won't or who are unable to, assimilate, which positions them as non-normative, at the peripheries of normative culture. This perspective will provide the basis for the next chapter.

Notes

1. The family formation of unrelated adults is not just evident in the sitcom genre. In her discussion of news anchor shows like *Good Morning America* (ABC 1975–present), Naficy Hamid (1989) identifies how the hosts are constructed in the text as a 'we' in the context of a substitute TV family. As she explains: 'Although members of these families are not related by blood, they continue to retain their basic heterosexual configuration, and they share in the common codes and values of the culture' (1989, 50).
2. *Friends* was added to Netflix UK in 2018, and according to Ofcom is currently the subscription service's most-streamed show.
3. Brenda is also the name of a popular lesbian dating app.
4. Throughout *Rules of Engagement*, homosexual connotations are made towards two male characters—wealthy real estate business owner, Russell, and his Indian personal assistant, Timir. In the final season, Russell forgets to renew Timir's work visa, and the pair get married.
5. A recent reworking of this notion that lesbian motherhood is culturally deemed incompatible with culture can be seen in the character of detective Miranda Hilmarson in *Top of the Lake: China Girl*. Although presented as heterosexual, Miranda's character is shaped as masculine, due to her extreme height and lack of the conventional signs of femininity, such as long hair, petite frame and make-up. In 'China Girl' (Season 2, Episode 1) two police colleagues sneer within her earshot: 'It's an actual woman by the way [laughter]'. This demonstrates an act of shaming the queer (Munt 2008). In addition to her masculine traits, Miranda is also involuntarily childless, and as the narrative reveals, she is one of the intended mother who has engaged a Thai surrogate to carry her genetic child. In the final episode, Miranda is shot in the stomach by a gunman, and is left brain dead in a coma. I propose this is a contemporary reiteration of the killing-off of the deviant queer. Miranda's queerness has excluded her from motherhood—she is not permitted a happy ending.
6. The exclusion of the lesbian body to enable a happy heterosexuality is also explored in Chapter 6, in relation to the lead character Robin in *Top of the Lake: China Girl*.
7. This surveillance of docile bodies can also be seen in *Top of the Lake: China Girl* and *The Handmaid's Tale*. The Thai surrogates in the former are kept in a secret room under constant supervision through CCTV, and the handmaids in the latter are imprisoned in the couple's home. As docile bodies, they are fed, given vitamins and regular check-ups, much like the surrogates discussed in this book. This form of surveillance in both shows also reflects the treatment of surrogates in India (Pande 2014).

8. It could also be argued that Goldie is showing qualities of both 'intensive' and 'good enough' mothering (Feasey 2015) by sacrificing her body and time to earn money through surrogacy to take care of her child.
9. Tor Folger's (2008) qualitative research on same-sex families in Norway identified a discourse of heterosexual romantic love—lifelong monogamy, the couple, heterosexual ritual—was core to how same-sex families shaped their family lives. According to his research one informant was surprised, he ended up in such a conventional life—with a family, living in the suburbs, talking over the fence, just like the other dads. As Folger argues: 'The traditional family life he lives represents a radical breach with earlier norms, and it may be seen as both conventional and unconventional at the same time' (2008, 144).

References

Ahmed, Sara. 2006. *Queer Phenomenology: Orientations, Objects, Others*. London: Routledge.

Ahmed, Sara. 2010. *The Promise of Happiness*. Durham: Duke University Press.

Allison, Christine. 1996. "The Making of a Bad Mother: A Lesbian Mother and Her Daughters." In *Between Monsters, Goddesses and Cyborgs: Feminist Confrontations with Science, Medicine and Cyberspace*, edited by Nina Lykke and Rosi Braidotti. London: Zed Books.

Aslinger, Ben. 2013. "'It's Not So Easy For Two Men To Be a Couple': Revisiting Gay Dating in *Will & Grace* and *Queer As Folk*." In *Queer Love in Film and Television: Critical Essays*, edited by Pamela Demory and Christopher Pullen. New York: Palgrave Macmillan.

Avila-Saavedra, Guillermo. 2009. "Nothing Queer About Queer Television: Televized Construction of Gay Masculinities." *Media Culture Society* 31 (1): 5–31.

Bartky, Sandra. 1991. *Femininity and Domination: Studies in the Phenomenology of Oppression*. London: Routledge.

Battles, Kathleen, and Wendy Hilton-Morrow. 2002. "Gay Characters in Conventional Spaces: Will and Grace and the Situation Comedy Genre." *Critical Studies in Media Communication* 19 (1): 87–105.

Battles, Kathleen, and Wendy Hilton-Morrow. 2015. *Sexual Identities and the Media*. New York: Routledge.

Becker, Ron. 2006. *Gay TV and Straight America*. New Brunswick, NJ: Rutgers University Press.

Benkov, Laura. 1994. *Reinventing the Family: The Emerging Story of Lesbian and Gay Parents*. New York: Crown Publishers.

Berlant, Lauren. 1994. "America, 'Fat,' the Fetus'." *Boundary 2* 21 (3): 145–195.

Berlant, Lauren. 2008. *The Female Complaint*. Durham: Duke University Press.
Berlant, Lauren. 2011. *Cruel Optimism*. Durham: Duke University Press.
Berlant, Lauren, and Michael Warner. 1998. "Sex in Public." *Critical Inquiry* 24 (2): 547–566.
Bogle, Donald. 2016. *Toms, Coons, Mulattoes, Mammies and Bucks: An Interpretative History of Blacks in American Films*, 5th ed. New York: Bloomsbury Academy.
Briggs, Laura. 2017. *How All Politics Became Reproductive Politics—From Welfare Reform to Foreclosure to Trump*. Berkeley: University of California Press.
Brook, Barbara. 1999. *Feminist Perspectives on the Body*. 1st ed. London: Routledge.
Brothers & Sisters. 1998–2004. Created by Jon Robin Baitz. TV Programme. Burbank, CA: Walt Disney.
Bruni, Frank. 1994. "Culture Stays Screen-Shy of Showing the Gay Kiss.' In *The Columbia Reader On Lesbian and Gay Men in Media, Society & Politics*, edited by Larry Gross and James D. Woods. New York: Columbia University Press.
Burke, Phyliss. 1993. *Family Values: Two Moms and Their Son*. New York: Random House.
Butler, Judith. 1990. *Gender Trouble*. New York: Routledge.
Butler, Judith. 1993. *Bodies That Matter: On the Discursive Limits of Sex*. London: Routledge.
Calhoun, Cheshire. 2000. *Feminism, Family, and the Politics of the Closet: Lesbian and Gay Displacement*. Oxford: Oxford University Press.
Cavalcante, André. 2014. "Anxious Displacements: The Representation of Gay Parenting on Modern Family and The New Normal and the Management of Cultural Anxiety." *Television & New Media* 1 (18): 454–471.
Charlebois, Justin. 2011. *Gender and the Construction of Hegemonic and Oppositional Femininities*. Lanham: Lexington.
Cheers. 1982–1993. Created by James Burrows, Glen Charles, Les Charles. TV Programme. New York: CBS/Paramount.
Cohen, Cathy J. 1997. "Punks, Bulldaggers, and Welfare Queens: The Radical Potential of Queer Politics?" *GLQ: A Journal of Lesbian and Gay Studies* 3 (4): 437–465.
Colebrook, Claire. 2003. *Gender*. London: Palgrave.
Connell, Raewyn, and James W. Messerschmidt. 2005. "Hegemonic Masculinity: Rethinking the Concept." *Gender & Society* 19 (6): 829–859.
Davis, Dana-Ain. 2009. "The Politics of Reproduction: The Troubling Case of Nadya Suleman and Assisted Reproductive Technology." *Transforming Anthropology* 17 (2): 105–116. https://doi.org/10.1111/j.1548-7466.2009.01061.x.

De Lauretis, Teresa. 1994. *The Practice of Love: Lesbian Sexuality and Perverse Desire*. Bloomington, IN: Indiana University Press.

Demory, Pamela, and Christopher Pullen. 2013. *Queer Love in Film and Television*. New York: Palgrave Macmillan.

Doty, Alexander. 1993. *Making Things Perfectly Queer: Interpreting Mass Culture*. Minneapolis: University of Minnesota Press.

Doty, Alexander. 2010. "Modern Family, Glee, and the Limits of Television Liberalism." *Flow Journal*, September 4. https://www.flowjournal.org/2010/09/modern-family-glee-and-limits-of-tv-liberalism/.

Douglas, Mary. 1968. "The Social Control of Cognition: Some Factors in Joke Recognition." *Man* 3: 361–376.

Dow, Bonnie. 1996. *Prime-Time Feminism: Television, Media Culture, and the Women's Movement Since 1970*. Philadelphia: University of Pennsylvania Press.

Dow, Bonnie. 2001. "Ellen, Television, and the Politics of Gay and Lesbian Visibility." *Critical Studies in Media Communication* 18 (2): 123–140.

Dowling, Robyn. 2003. "Femininity, Place and Commodities: A Retail Case Study." *Antipode* 25: 295–319.

Duggan, Lisa. 2002. "The New Homonormativity: The Sexual Politics of Neoliberalism." In *Materializing Democracy*, edited by R. Russ Castronovo and Dana D. Nelson. Durham: Duke University Press.

Duits, Linda, and Pauline van Romondt Vis. 2009. "Girls Make Sense: Girls, Celebrities, and Identities." *European Journal of Cultural Studies* 12 (1): 41–58.

Dyer, Richard. 1977. *White*. London: Routledge.

Dyer, Richard. 1993. *The Matter of Images: Essays on Representations*. London: Routledge.

Dyer, Richard. 2012. *Culture of Queers*. London: Routledge.

Edelman, Lee. 2003. *No Future: Queer Theory and the Death Drive*. Durham: Duke University Press.

Evans, Mary. 2003. *Love: An Unromantic Discussion*. Cambridge: Polity Press.

Feasey, Rebecca. 2008. *Masculinity and Popular Television*. Edinburgh: Edinburgh University Press.

Feasey, Rebecca. 2013. "From Soap Opera to Reality Programming: Examining Motherhood, Motherwork and the Maternal Role on Popular Television." *Imaginations: Journal of Cross-Cultural Image Studies* 4 (2): 25–46.

Feasey, Rebecca. 2015. *Mothers on Mothers: Maternal Readings of Popular Television*. Edinburgh: Edinburgh University Press.

Feasey, Rebecca. 2017. "Good, Bad or Just Good Enough: Representations of Motherhood and the Maternal Role on the Small Screen." *Studies in the Maternal* 9 (1): 5, 1–31. https://doi.org/10.16995/sim.234.

Fejes, Fred. 2000. "Making a Gay Masculinity." *Critical Studies in Media Communication*, 17 (1): 113–116.

Fejes, Fred, and Petrich, Kevin. 2013. "Invisibility, Homophobia and Heterosexism: Lesbians, Gays and the Media." *Review and Criticism*, 10 (4): 396–422.

Folger, Tom. 2008. "Queer Nuclear Families? Reproducing and Transgressing Heteronormativity." *Journal of Homosexuality* 54 (1–2): 124–149. http://dx.doi.org/10.1080/00918360801952028.

Foucault, Michel. 1977. *Discipline and Punish: The Birth of the Prison*. London: Penguin.

Foucault, Michel. 1984. "Of Other Spaces: Utopias and Heterotopias." Translated from *Architecture, Mouvement, Continuité* 5: 46–49.

Foucault, Michel. 1998. *The History of Sexuality: The Will to Knowledge: The Will to Knowledge*, vol. 1. New ed. London: Penguin.

Freud, Sigmund. 1977. *On Sexuality*, 1st ed. London: Penguin.

Friedan, Betty. 2010. *The Feminine Mystique*. London: Penguin Classics.

Friends. 1992–2004. Created by David Crane, Marta Kauffman. TV Programme. New York: NBC.

Frutkin, Anne. 1995. "Family Outings." *Advocate* 62: 30–31.

Gibbs, Anna. 2001. "Contagious Feelings: Pauline Hanson and the Epidemiology of Affect." *Australian Humanities Review* 24.

Gilson, Duane. 2016. "'Homonormativity' and Its Discontents." *The Gay & Lesbian Review*, January–February: 22–24.

GLAAD. 2018. "Accelerating Acceptance 2018." https://www.glaad.org/publications/accelerating-acceptance-2018. Accessed February 1, 2019.

Glee. 2009–2014. Created by Ian Brennan, Brad Falchuk, Ryan Murphy. TV Programme. Los Angeles, CA: Fox.

Goltz, Dustin Bradley. 2011. *Queer Temporalities in Gay Male Representation*, 1st ed. London: Routledge.

Gorton, Kristyn. 2009. *Media Audiences*. Edinburgh: Edinburgh University Press.

Grey's Anatomy. Created by Shonda Rhimes. 2005–present. TV Programme. New York: ABC.

Gross, Larry, and James Woods. 1999. *The Columbia Reader of Lesbians and Gay Men in Media, Society & Politics*. New York: Columbia University Press.

Halberstam, Judith. 1998. *Female Masculinity*. Durham: Duke University Press.

Halberstam, Judith. 2011. *The Queer Art of Failure*. Durham: Duke University Press.

Halberstam, Judith. 2013. *Gaga Feminism: Sex, Gender and the End of Normal*. Boston: Beacon Press.

Hilton-Morrow, Wendy. 2015. *Sexual Identities and the Media*, 1st ed. New York: Routledge.

Hughey, Matthew. 2014. *The White Savior Film: Content, Critics, and Consumption*. Philadelphia: Temple University Press.

Jones, Terry, and Robert Staples. 1985. "Culture, Ideology and Black Television Images." *The Black Scholar* 16 (3): 10–20.

Kaplan, Anne. 1998. *Film Noir*. London: British Film Institute.

Katz Rothman, Barbara. 2005. *Weaving a Family: Untangling Race and Adoption*. Boston: Beacon Press.

Kinnick, Katherine. 2009. "Media Morality Tales and the Politics of Motherhood." In *Mommy Angst: Motherhood in American Popular Culture*, edited by Anne Hall and Mardia Bishop. Santa Barbara, CA: Praeger/ABC-CLIO.

Kristeva, Julia. 1980. *Desire in Language: A Semiotic Approach to Literature and Art*. New York: Columbia University Press.

Kuhn, Annette. 1992. *Women's Pictures: Feminism and Cinema*. 2nd ed. London: Verso.

Kunze, Peter. 2013. "Family Guys: Same-Sex Parenting and Masculinity in Modern Family." In *Queer Love in Film and Television: Critical Essays*, edited by Pamela Demory and Christopher Pullen. New York: Palgrave Macmillan.

Lam, Carla. 2015. *New Reproductive Technologies and Disembodiment*, 1st ed. Abingdon: Routledge.

LaVecchia, Christina. 2011. "Of Peerenting, Trophy Wives, and Effeminate Men: Modern. Family's Surprisingly Conservative Remediation of the Family Sitcom Genre." *Harlot: A Revealing Look at the Arts of Persuasion* 6. http://harlotofthearts.org/index.php/harlot/article/view/85/65.

Lee, Pei-Wen, and Michaela Meyer. 2010. "'We All Have Feelings for Our Girlfriends:' Progressive (?) Representations of Lesbian Lives on the The L Word." *Sexuality & Culture* 14 (3): 234–250.

Lehr, Valerie. 1999. *Queer Family Values: Debunking the Myth of the Nuclear Family*. Philadelphia: Temple University Press.

Lewin, Ellen. 1993. *Lesbian Mothers: Accounts of Gender in American Culture*. New York: Cornell University Press.

Lewis, Ruth, and Judith Scanlon. 2016. "Whose sexuality is it anyway? Women's experiences of viewing lesbians on screen." *Feminist Media Studies* 17 (6): 1005–1021.

Linneman, Thomas J. 2008. "How Do You Solve a Problem Like Will Truman?: The Feminization of Gay Masculinities on Will & Grace." *Men and Masculinities* 10 (5): 583–603. https://doi.org/10.1177/1097184x06291918.

Lockyer, Sharon, and Michael Pickering. 2008. "You Must Be Joking: The Sociological Critique of Humour and Comic Media." *Sociology Compass* 2 (3): 808–820. https://doi.org/10.1111/j.1751-9020.2008.00108.x.

Lucas, Jennifer, and Amber B. Raley. 2006. "Stereotype or Success?" *Journal of Homosexuality* 51 (2): 19–38.

Martin, Biddy. 1997. *Femininity Played Straight: Significance of Being Lesbian*, 1st ed. London: Routledge.

McCormick, Adrienne. 2010. "Supermothers on Film: or Maternal Melodrama in the Twenty-First Century." In *21st Century Motherhood: Experience, Identity, Policy, Agency*, edited by Andrea O'Reilly. New York: Columbia University Press.

McKee, Alan. 1996. "A Kiss Is Just…" *Australian Journal of Communication* 23 (2): 51–72.

McNicholas Smith, Kate, and Imogen Tyler. 2017. "Lesbian Brides: Post-Queer Popular Culture." *Feminist Media Studies* 17 (3): 315–331.

Mills, Brett. 2005. *Television Sitcom*. London: British Film Institute.

Mills, Brett. 2009. *The Sitcom*. Edinburgh: Edinburgh University Press.

Modern Family. 2009–present. Created by Steven Levitan, Christopher Lloyd. TV Programme. Los Angeles, CA: ABC.

Morgan, Michael. 1982. "Television and Adolescents' Sex Role Stereotypes: A Longitudinal Study." *Journal of Personality and Social Psychology* 43 (5): 947–955.

Moritz, Marguerite. 1987. "Coming Out Stories: The Creation of Lesbian Images on Prime Time TV." Paper presented at the Speech Communication Association Convention, Boston.

Moritz, Marguerite. 1999. "Old Strategies for New Texts: How American Television Is Creating and Treating Lesbian Characters." In *The Columbia Reader On Lesbian and Gay Men in Media, Society & Politics*, edited by Larry Gross and James D. Woods. New York: Columbia University Press.

Muñoz, José. 2007. *Cruising Utopia: The Then and There of Queer Futurity*. New York: New York University Press.

Muñoz, José. 2009. *Cruising Utopia: The Then and There of Queer Futurity*. New York: New York University Press.

Munt, Sally R. 1998. *Butch-Femme: Inside Lesbian Genders*. London: Cassell.

Munt, S. 2008. *Queer Attachments: The Cultural Politics of Shame*, 1st ed. Aldershot: Ashgate.

My So-Called Life. 1994–1995. Created by Winnie Holzman. TV Programme. Los Angeles, CA: ABC.

Naficy, Hamid. 1989. "Television Intertextuality and the Discourse of the Nuclear Family." *Journal of Film and Video* 41 (4): 42–59.

Nelson, Fiona. 2007. "Mother Tongues: The Discursive Journeys of Lesbian and Heterosexual Women into Motherhood." *Journal of GLBT Family Studies* 3: 223–265.

Nelson, Fiona. 2009. *In the Other Room: Entering the Culture of Motherhood*. Halifax, NS: Fernwood Publishing.

Oliver, Kelly. 2012. *Knock Me Up, Knock Me Down*. New York: Columbia University Press.

Orange Is the New Black. 2013–present. Created by Jenji Kohan. TV Programme. Santa Monica, CA: Lionsgate Television.

Packer, Vin. 1952. *Spring Fire*. New York: Gold Medal.

Pande, Amrita. 2014. *Wombs in Labor: Transnational Commercial Surrogacy in India*. New York: Columbia University Press.

Park, Shelley. 2006. "Adoptive Maternal Bodies: A Queer Paradigm for Rethinking Mothering?" *Hypatia* 21 (1): 201–226.

Park, Shelley. 2014. *Mothering Queerly, Queering Motherhood*. New York: State University of New York Press.

Probyn, Elspeth. 2005. *Blush: Faces of Shame*. Minneapolis: University of Minnesota Press.

Pugh, Tison. 2018. *Queer Fantasises of the American Family Sitcom*. New Brunswick, NJ: Rutgers University Press.

Queer Voices. 2016. "One Million Moms: New Normal Got Cancelled Because of Our Persistence." *Huffington Post*. February 2, 2015. http://www.huffingtonpost.com/2013/05/16/one-million-moms-new-normal-cancellation-_n_3287973.html.

Radicalesbians. 1970. "The Woman Identified Woman." Atlanta Lesbian Feminist Archives: Know, Inc. Accessed January 1, 2016. http://library.duke.edu/digitalcollections/wlmpc_wlmms01011_wlmms010110010/.

Rich, Adrienne. 1980. "Compulsory Heterosexuality and Lesbian Existence." *Signs: Journal of Women in Culture and Society* 5 (4): 631–660.

Richardson, Diane. 2005. "Claiming Citizenship? Sexuality, Citizenship and Lesbian Feminist Theory." In *Thinking Straight: New Work in Critical Heterosexuality Studies*, edited by Chrys Ingraham. New York: Routledge.

Roberts, Dorothy. 1996. "Race and the New Reproduction." *Faculty Scholarship at Penn Law*. 1154.

Roof, Judith. 1998. "1970s Lesbian Feminism Meets 1990s Butch/Femme." In *Butch/Femme: Inside Lesbian Gender*, edited by Sally R. Munt. London: Cassell.

Rubin, Gayle. 2011. *Deviations: A Gayle Rubin Reader*. New York: Duke University Press.

Rules of Engagement. 2007–2013. "Les-Bro." Season 5, Episode 8. Directed by Ted Wass. Written by Tom Hertz, Gloria Calderon Kellett. TV Programme. November 8, 2010. New York: CBS.

Rules of Engagement. 2007–2013. "Uh-oh It's Magic." Season 5, Episode 14. Directed by Gail Mancuso. Written by Tom Hertz, Lance Whinery. TV Programme. January 3, 2011. New York: CBS.

Rules of Engagement. 2007–2013. "Beating the System." Season 5, Episode 20. Directed by Tom Hertz. Written by Becky Mann, Audra Sielaff. TV Programme. April 7, 2011. New York: CBS.

Rules of Engagement. 2007–2013. "100th." Season 7, Episode 13. Directed and written by Tom Hertz. TV programme. May 20, 2013. New York: CBS.

Schulman, Sarah. 1998. *Stagestruck: Theatre, AIDS, and the Marketing of Gay America*. Durham: Duke University Press.

Scodari, Christine. 1995. "Possession, Attraction, and the Thrill of The Chase: Gendered Myth Making in Film and Television Comedy of the Sexes." *Critical Studies in Mass Communication* 12: 23–29.

Sedgwick, Eve Kosofsky. 2008. *Epistemology of the Closet.* Berkeley: University of California Press.

Seidman, Steven. 2004. *Beyond the Closet: The Transformation of Gay and Lesbian Life.* New York: Routledge.

Sex and the City. 1998–2004. Created by Darren Star. TV Programme. New York: HBO.

SmithBattle, Lee. 2013. "Reducing the Stigmatization of Teen Mothers." *MCN: The American Journal of Maternal/Child Nursing* 38(4): 235–241; quiz: 242-3. https://doi.org/10.1097/nmc.0b013e3182836bd4.

Sourbut, Elizabeth. 1996. "Gynogenesis: A Lesbian Appropriation of Reproductive Technologies." In *Between Monsters, Goddesses and Cyborgs: Feminist Confrontations with Science, Medicine and Cyberspace*, edited by Nina Lykke, and Rosi Braidotti. London: Zed Books.

Stacey, Jackie. 1993. *Star Gazing: Hollywood Cinema and Female Spectatorship*, 1st ed. New York: Routledge.

Sullivan, Andrew. 1995. *Virtually Normal.* New York: Vintage.

The Birdcage. 1996. Directed by Mike Nichols. Written by Jean Poiret, Elaine May. Film. Beverly Hills, CA: United Artists.

The Fosters. 2013–present. Created by Bradley Bredeweg, Peter Paige. TV Programme. Burbank, CA: Freeform.

The Kids Are All Right. 2010. Directed by Lisa Cholodenko. Written by Lisa Cholodenko, Stuart Blumberg. Film. Los Angeles, CA: Focus Features.

The New Normal. 2012–2013. Created by Elodie Keene, Max Winkler, Ryan Murphy. TV Programme. New York: NBC.

The New Normal. 2012–2013. "Pilot." Season 1. Episode 1. Directed by Ryan Murphy. Written by Ryan Murphy, Ali Adler. TV Programme. September 10, 2012. New York: NBC.

The New Normal. 2012–2013. "Sofa's Choice." Season 1. Episode 2. Directed by Ryan Murphy. Written by Ryan Murphy, Ali Adler. TV Programme. September 11, 2012. New York: NBC.

The New Normal. 2012–2013. "Baby Clothes." Season 1. Episode 3. Directed by Ryan Murphy. Written by Ryan Murphy, Ali Adler. TV Programme. September 18, 2012. New York: NBC.

The New Normal. 2012–2013. "Obama Mama." Season 1. Episode 4. Directed by Scott Ellis. Written by Ryan Murphy, Ali Adler. TV Programme. September 25, 2012. New York: NBC.

The New Normal. 2012–2013. "Bryanzilla." Season 1. Episode 6. Directed by Ryan Murphy. Written by Ryan Murphy, Ali Adler. TV Programme. October 9, 2012. New York: NBC.

The New Normal. 2012–2013. "Stay-at-home Dad." Season 1. Episode 13. Directed by Bradley Buecker. Written by Ryan Murphy, Ali Adler. TV Programme. January 15, 2013. New York: NBC.

The New Normal. 2012–2013. "Blood, Sweat and Fears." Season 1. Episode 15. Directed by Elodie Keene. Written by Ryan Murphy, Ali Adler. TV Programme. March 19, 2013. New York: NBC.

The New Normal. 2012–2013. "Dairy Queen." Season 1. Episode 19. Directed by Bradley Buecker. Written by Ryan Murphy, Ali Adler. TV Programme. January 29, 2013. New York: NBC.

The New Normal. 2012–2013. "The Big Day." Season 1. Episode 22. Directed by Max Winkler. Written by Ryan Murphy, Ali Adler. TV Programme. April 2, 2013. New York: NBC.

The Simpsons. 1989–present. Created by Matt Groening. TV Programme. Los Angeles, CA: 20th Television.

Thirtysomething. 1987–1991. "Strangers." Season 3. Episode 6. Directed by Peter O'Fallon. Written by Marshall Herskovitz, Edward Zwick. TV Programme. New York: ABC.

Throsby, Karen. 2004. *When IVF Fails: Feminism, Infertility and the Negotiation of Normal*. Basingstoke: Palgrave.

Townsend, Megan. 2018. "GLAAD's 'Where We Are on TV' Report Shows Television Telling More LGBTQ Stories Than Ever." October 25. https://www.glaad.org/blog/glaads-where-we-are-tv-report-shows-television-telling-more-lgbtq-stories-ever.

True Blood. 2008–2014. Created by Alan Ball. TV Programme. New York: HBO.

Tyler, Imogen. 2008. "Why the Maternal Now?" Published by the Department of Sociology, Lancaster University, Lancaster LA1 4YT, UK. http://www.lancs.ac.uk/fass/sociology/papers/tylerwhythematernalnow.pdf.

Ugly Betty. 2006–2010. Created by Fernando Gaitain. TV Programme. Los Angeles, CA: ABC.

Villarejo, Amy. 2003. *Lesbian Rule: Cultural Criticism and the Value of Desire*. Durham: Duke University Press.

Walters, Suzanna. 2001. *All the Rage: The Story of Gay Visibility in America*. Chicago: University of Chicago Press.

Walters, Suzanna. 2012. "The Kids Are All Right But The Lesbians Aren't: Queer Kinship in US Culture." *Sexuality* 15 (8): 917–933. https://doi.org/10.1177/1363460712459311.

Warner, Michael. 1999. *The Trouble with Normal*. Cambridge, MA: Harvard University Press.

Ward, Jane. 2008. *Respectably Queer: Diversity Culture in LGBT Activist Organizations*. Nashville: Vanderbilt University Press.

White, Patricia. 1999. *Uninvited: Classical Hollywood Cinema and Lesbian Representability*, New ed. Bloomington: Indiana University Press.

Williams, Linda. 1991. "Film Bodies: Gender, Genre, and Excess." *Film Quarterly* 44 (4): 2–13.

Will & Grace. 1998–2006. Created by David Kohan, Max Mutchnick. TV Programme. New York: NBC.

Wittig, Monique. 1992. *The Straight Mind: And Other Essays*. Boston: Beacon Press.

Wolfe, Susan J., and Lee Ann Roripaugh. 2006. "The (In)visible Lesbian: Anxieties of Representation in the L Word." In *Reading 'The L Word': Outing Contemporary Television*, edited by Kim Akass and Janet McCabe. London: Tauris.

Young, Iris. 1984. "Pregnant Embodiment: Subjectivity and Alienation." *The Journal of Medicine and Philosophy* 9 (1): 45–62.

Zeller-Jacques, Martin. 2011. "'Challenging and Alternative': Screening Queer Girls on Channel 4." In *Women on Screen: Feminism and Femininity in Visual Culture*, edited by Melanie Waters. London: Palgrave Macmillan.

CHAPTER 4

Infertile Bodies: Rescuing Infertility Through the Heterosexual Love Plot

The previous chapter explored how the homosexual and lesbian characters in *The New Normal* and *Rules of Engagement* transform into a normative position through the employment of 'happiness scripts' (Ahmed 2010, 91) which I have argued, through characterisation, narrative, acting and the script, embody conventions of heteronormativity. In this chapter, the concept of *queer straightness* that was employed previously to explore the representation of homosexual and lesbian characters will be transposed into a *straight queerness*. This concept has been constructed to describe the straightening (Ahmed 2010) of heterosexual-identified characters that I argue are situated in a non-normative position by being infertile.

Both *queer straightness* and *straight queerness* are concepts that have been formed to aid the exploration of normalising techniques, which I propose emerge in the narrative structures under analysis, in relation to creating a family through surrogacy. This will be achieved in this chapter by examining how the lead childless heterosexual female characters in *Baby Mama* and *Rules of Engagement* are depicted as being non-normative. I propose that both characters are, through the straightening narrative device of heteronormative love and family, *rescued* from their infertility, *and* any possibility of being culturally recognised as a lesbian subject. Both characters' infertility is cured—they discover they

L. Le Vay, *Surrogacy and the Reproduction of Normative Family on TV*, Palgrave Studies in Science and Popular Culture,
https://doi.org/10.1007/978-3-030-17570-2_4

are pregnant naturally when their surrogates go into labour. I argue that this transformation from infertile to fertile repositions them within the normative.

Straight queerness was introduced in brief by Alexander Doty (1993) in his discussion of the use of the term *queer* to 'describe a wide range of impulses and cultural expressions' (1993, 2). This diversification of the term from its original identification within queer politics also supports Judith Butler's (1993) call for the term to be 'redeployed, twisted, queered from prior usage and in the direction of urgent and expanding political purposes' (1993, 228). Although Butler claimed that 'exposing the naturalized status of heterosexuality' (1993, 231) wouldn't necessarily lead to its subversion, to view queer as resistance to the normative, by being positioned as non-normative, best explains its mobilisation in this chapter. As Lee Edelman (2004) states, queer is a verb term that can describe anyone 'failing to comply' (2004, 17). Therefore, queer as a tool to explore the non-normative will be employed as the primary analytical lens in this chapter.

Cathy J. Cohen's (1997) call for a coalition politics also plays a central role in these discussions as she argues that queer politics has not destabilised categories of identity but has in fact reinforced them through strengthening the divisions between heterosexuality 'and everything "queer"' (1997, 438). Cohen identified that the impact of power on the identity of marginalised subjects on both sides of the hetero/homo binary has been left unexamined. She also claims that New York LGBTQ organisation Queer Nation's activism against heterosexual oppression during the 1990s failed to acknowledge that non-normative practices of family and reproduction *also* exist within those who are labelled heterosexual. Cohen proposed that heterosexuality should not be viewed as monolithic, and that heterosexual subjects are also regulated and excluded by dominant heterosexual culture,[1] who, like lesbians and gays, can also be viewed as gender deviants by failing to conform to traditional gender roles (Calhoun 2000).

Therefore, this chapter aims to introduce new ways of thinking about what is positioned as non-normative in popular culture, which includes the 'normative category of heterosexuality' (Cohen 1997, 439). Explaining how and why the construction of infertile bodies in these texts, despite being white and heterosexual, are positioned in opposition to norms will accomplish this. However, as will be explored, the prospect of occupying this oppositional space for transformational potential, to enable the lesbian, the uncoupled, and women coping with infertility to emerge in the narrative, is shut down. This is demonstrated through the narrative facilitating the transition of infertile to fertile—and in *Baby Mama*, the protagonist's narrative journey from single to couple. Therefore, I have extended Doty's term of ***straight queerness*** to describe the effect of these normalising devices, and to show how the construction of infertility in these texts share an affinity with the non-normative (the queer) by being positioned at the margins of social norms.

The concept of *straight queerness* will be developed primarily through the engagement of queer and feminist work on compulsory heterosexuality, lesbian existence, emotions and affect. This body of work also underpins a queer reading of *Baby Mama*, led by a 'masculinization of motherhood' (Lam 2015, 33), a key theme that has emerged as noteworthy in the audience data. This reading has been implemented to further illustrate how characters affected by infertility have been positioned as non-normative.

By exploring this notion of masculinisation, I argue that the relationship between the single childless character Kate, and her surrogate, Angie, can be read as sexually ambiguous. This reading demonstrates how the love plot performs as a straightening device, as a form of rescue, not just from infertility but also the possibility of lesbian sexuality, the narrative closure returning the female characters to their proper place—the home, motherhood and family (Kuhn 1992; Moritz 1987, 1999; Walker 1982). This approach also reflects an openness to possible erotic nuances in texts which helps to explore a heterosexism that exists at the core of contemporary television (Gantz in Thomas 2000; Sedgwick 2008).

This chapter unfolds over three sections. "You're Not a Real Woman" aims to explain this affinity of heterosexual infertility and lesbian subject position at the margins of dominant social norms. "There's Nothing Queer About It" offers a queer reading of the texts in relation to gender norms and compulsory heterosexuality, and "Someday My Prince Will Come" will illustrate how the heterosexual love plot rescues the infertile characters by making them fertile.

You're Not a Real Woman

You're not a real woman until you've had a child.

(Laura, non-mothers focus group, 2015)

Characters Audrey in *Rules of Engagement* and Kate in *Baby Mama* are both childless, involuntarily. Due to the failure of IVF, they turn to surrogacy. Audrey is married, and Kate is single. Both are depicted as straight. Kate employs a surrogacy agency and uses donor sperm. Audrey's husband's friend, Brenda, who is a lesbian, offers her surrogacy services. Audrey and Kate are white, successful middle-class women in their late thirties. Audrey is a magazine editor, Kate a VP of a grocery chain. Both narratives infer that they have put their careers ahead of starting a family. *Baby Mama's* opening scene shows Kate in her workplace. Her voiceover discloses: 'when people got pregnant, I got promotions'. This reflects the common character trope of the childless career woman, which also emerges in film *Baby Boom* (1987) and in TV series *Ally McBeal* (Fox 1997–2002). As explored in Chapter 2, this hunger for a child (Davitz 1984; Hewlett 2002) has struck a growing number of professional women who have the funds to explore fertility options such as IVF and surrogacy, who are now being reflected in popular media characterisations, such as the childless characters in *Baby Mama* and *Rules of Engagement*. Due to struggling with an infertility diagnosis, I propose they are depicted as unhappy failures—positioned as non-normative. Such feelings have been identified as common among women whose treatment has been unsuccessful, a sense of failure which drives the discourse of desperateness which is amplified in media narratives (Franklin 1990; Throsby 2004).

The baby shower scene in *Rules of Engagement* (Season 6, Episode 16: 'Audrey's Shower') emerged as significant in the audience data and will provide the focus for this section. This scene shows Audrey as being isolated from what is culturally marked as a heterosexual ritual/life milestone for women (Griffin 2009). When she stands to address her guests, the surrogate Brenda announces that the baby is kicking. Audrey's friends turn their backs on her and face the surrogate, an action that indicates a public shaming of the isolated subject, through a bodily level, who is left feeling out-of-place and insecure in one's surroundings (Gorton 2009; Probyn 2005). Laura (non-mothers focus group) detected the bodily tension between Audrey and Brenda, and identified Audrey's positioning as non-normative:

> There was only one thing that struck me that had some truth in it, and it was at the shower thing, when she [Audrey] tries to stand up to talk and Brenda goes, "It's kicking!" and everyone's attention turns to her, and

> you think, shit, it must feel really weird, as you know... to not be able to have... she must feel so jealous, but you have to contain jealousy and it's like, not healthy is it, it's storing up all that emotion, you gotta let it out, she probably wanted to scream, and say "but you're all here for me! It's my baby!"
>
> (Laura, non-mothers focus group, 2015)

What Laura is demonstrating through her response to the characterisation and the narrative in this scene is what cognitive film theorist Murray Smith (1995) calls 'emotional stimulation' (1995, 97). This is when the viewer observes the behaviour of a fictional person, and projects themselves into the scene and their situation, which enables the viewer to guess the emotions the character is experiencing. As Laura described: 'she must feel so jealous', 'it must feel really weird', 'she probably wanted to scream!' Kirstyn Gorton (2009) explains: 'In the cognitive model, spectators relate to the emotions the characters experience rather than identify with the characters themselves' (2009, 78). Laura did not see an image of herself reflected back through the character of Audrey, but was, instead, able to empathise with, or relate to, the *emotions* the character is shown as experiencing, constructed through scene sequencing, composition and acting, by the sitcom writers and directors (Carroll 2005). Drawing on Greg Smith (1999), this baby shower scene which Laura described had 'struck' her, illustrates emotion markers that have been engineered in the text—textual cues that aim to elicit 'brief moments of emotion' (in Gorton 2009, 80). It was up to Laura, as the viewer, to accept or decline the text's invitation to feel (Geraghty 2003). She accepted.

In this baby shower scene, and in relation to how emotions are constructed in the texts, I argue, drawing on Sara Ahmed (2010), that the foetus is being depicted as an object embedded with affective value, promising happiness before it's been experienced. 'Everyone's attention' turns to the surrogate and the kicking foetus, which illustrates how, as a 'happy object', the foetus is encircled by feelings of happiness by being 'what good feeling is directed toward' (2010, 25). As has been identified through this thesis, the goal in the narratives is to get the baby and become a mother, through the intervention of the disciplinary practice of reproductive technologies (Farquhar 1996; Sawicki 1992). As Ahmed argues, objects are not just physical or material, such as the foetus in this context, but 'anything that we imagine might lead us to happiness, including objects in the sense of values, practice, styles, as well as aspirations' (2010, 29). Within this discussion, this describes the aspiration of motherhood and the creation of normative family. By recognising that Audrey was 'storing up' negative emotions in response to the happy feelings directed to the surrogate's fertile body, Laura points to how shame is employed to differentiate the two bodies, which underscores the polarised non-normative/normative positions. What is also evident in this scene is how divisions have been formed between the women through tension—fertility, infertility—at an event that can be painful for women enduring infertility. As Margarete Sandelowski (1990) has highlighted through her work exploring fictional narratives with infertile respondents, the baby shower is a ritual that stirs difficult feelings of exclusion and hostility. Sandelowski recalls from her discussion sessions with her participants that they 'described similar feelings of coercion in maintaining a façade of cheer for other women's pregnancies and guilt over the feelings of rage and envy that lay behind the façade' (1990, 36). Although in this narrative the surrogate Brenda is carrying Audrey's genetic child, the emotional structure of the scene is similar. What is interesting about this scene is that the heterosexual character is positioned as non-normative, and the lesbian as normative. This twist, however, is temporary—the disruption stage in the narrative. The resolution/narrative closure is Audrey falling pregnant naturally, and the lesbian surrogate happily relinquishing the child. This conforms to heterosexist notions of normative motherhood, to be discussed further on.

Audrey is isolated through what can be read as a public shaming of her inability to carry her own foetus, witnessed by the guests at her baby shower in the text *and* by the individual viewer (Ahmed 2010; Probyn 2005; Sedgwick 2003). Her body language displays an affective embodiment of shame (Fig. 4.1)—her eyes look down, she holds her arms close to her body—she looks uncomfortable and uncertain (Ahmed 2010; Sedgwick 2003). As seen in Elspeth Probyn's (2005) observations on TV and shame, I propose that the emotion constructed in this scene articulates a shared shameful moment, aired for literally 'all to see' (in Gorton 2009, 61). As Beverley Skeggs (1997) identifies: 'Shame involves recognition of the judgment of others and awareness of social norms: one measures oneself against the standards established by others' (1997, 122). Paula's (non-mothers focus group) response to this scene reflects this: 'It's that part of motherhood that they miss out on,

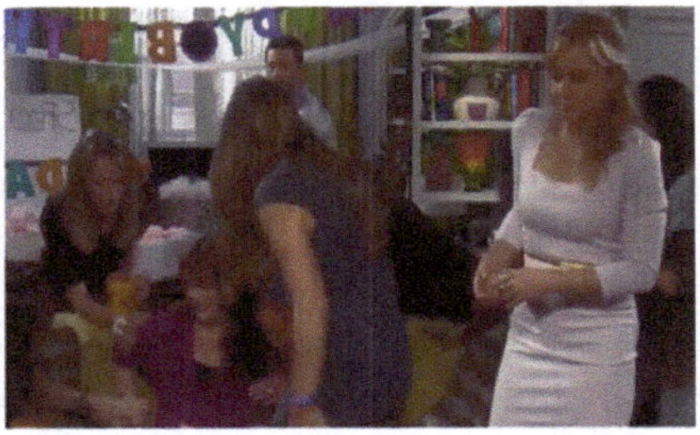

Fig. 4.1 *Rules of Engagement*, Season 6, Episode 16, "Audrey's Shower", directed by Ted Wass, aired May 17, 2012 on CBS, accessed July 22, 2017, https://www.pinterest.co.uk/aseals23/rules-of-engagement/

getting all the attention, it must be really difficult'. As viewers in this moment, both Laura and Paula were able to share this shameful moment as they were able to project themselves into the scene and empathise with the character's emotions. This demonstrates the effectiveness of the emotional engagement between the viewer and the screen (Gorton 2008, 2009). As Probyn (2005) argues, it's not just what affect *is*, it's also what it *does*. In this scene, shame alienates Audrey in the space, and positions her on the outside of social norms. She is depicted—and read by the participants—as unhappy in contrast to the happy surrogate. This is a technique that employs the happy/sad binary that steers the sitcom formula, which also illustrates its convention of mocking vulnerable subjects (Mills 2009).

While Audrey can be read as *feeling* shame through being positioned as non-normative, it can also be argued that she is *being* shamed through these genre devices. Audrey has become 'out of line with an affective community' (Ahmed 2010, 41) by disturbing normative heterosexual ritual. Therefore, it can be proposed that happy heterosexuality is bound up in the ability to reproduce. This has been identified as a dominant theme in the audience data, as Laura (non-mothers focus group) stated, somewhat annoyed by how Audrey is shown in this scene: 'You're not a real woman until you've had a child'. Paula (non-mothers focus group) and Carla (mixed mothers focus group) both identified the categorisation of 'woman' and value in relation to motherhood:

> Paula: There's this kind of underlying thing that in order to be a woman, you have to have a baby.
>
> Carla: It creates so much unhappiness actually, because what it says is you're not really trying, and you're not valid if you don't have a child.
>
> (Paula and Carla, non-mothers, and mixed mothers focus groups, 2015)

As Barbara Brook (1999) highlights: 'In numerous discourses, to be a "real woman" is to be "fertile"' (1999, 46). This belief has been widely contested by feminists as it posits the ideology that to be a real woman one has to be able to conceive, naturally. For example, Adrienne Rich (1980) argues that throughout history, childless women—alongside single women and widows—are seen as deviants, as they aren't assuming the natural role expected of women, as wives, mothers, caretakers. Psychologists Pamela Ashurst and Zaida Hall (1989) have identified anxieties in relation to feelings of incompleteness and motherhood, in their work with distressed women, arguing that: 'When a woman has a child, she confirms for herself and others that she is a complete woman, fertile and capable of the biological task of creating and perpetuating life' (1989, 97). This suggests that to be infertile (or childless by choice) is unnatural, and as Laura, Paula and Carla have all recognised in their interpretation of the texts, is to be *less* of a woman. This discourse echoes the essentialist hierarchical Cartesian binary of nature/culture, which aligns women's bodies with reproduction. Ellen Lewin (1993) argues in her discussion of the range of feminist debates on motherhood and women's oppression: 'All of these perspectives tend to conflate motherhood and womanhood, as though they were interchangeable, mutually defining, as though the status of woman could be entirely understood with respect to the meaning of motherhood' (1993, 5). Rachel's (non-mothers focus group) reading of how the childless characters were situated in the surrogacy narrative was enlightening:

> I think that's to do with a societal pressure, like, back to, again, you're not a real woman until you've had a child, so you're somehow broken. You've tried everything, but you're still broken. The surrogacy thing is just a stepping-stone to you becoming a real woman. And if it works out [natural pregnancy] then surrogacy's forgotten. At the end, you've got a baby, that's the main thing. I think that's what all those shows are about.
>
> (Rachel, non-mothers focus group, 2015)

By deciphering the dominant encoding in the texts as implying that a woman with fertility concerns isn't viewed as 'a real woman until you've had a child', this echoes Carla Lam's (2015) description of a 'reproductive misfit' (2015, 112). Lam claims this term applies to women who, due to their infertility, are viewed by dominant culture as oddities, who, if they wish to become mothers, have to utilise reproductive technologies to transcend the limitations of their bodies. This term was extended from disability theorist Rosemarie Garland-Thomson's (2011) concept of *misfitting*, which she employed to describe how vulnerable subjects struggle to interact with their environment on a daily basis, the 'dynamic encounter between flesh and world' which produces 'a coherent narrative of how inferiority is assigned and literal marginalization takes place' (2011, 592, 601). Misfitting explains whether such encounters are either harmonious, or disjunctive. To fit or misfit is not fixed, but changes over time, in relation to changes of body and environment, and barriers which are created through social attitudes and identity formations (Alcoff 2006; Garland-Thomson 2011; Lam 2015).

Further to the concept of misfitting—'broken' due to infertility—what can also be identified in Rachel's response is a description of the desire for the object of the genetic child, as has been discussed in this chapter , which can be both enabling and disabling. Enabling in the sense that it brings the 'woman' closer to the object that signifies the promise of happiness, driving her forward, and disabling in the sense that it gets in the way of happiness, by being cruelly optimistic (Ahmed 2010; Berlant 2011). Rachel's comment: 'If it works out then surrogacy is forgotten' implies that the representation of a baby born through surrogacy is not the ideal outcome. As also commented on by Charlie (non-mothers focus group): 'It [the natural pregnancy] makes surrogacy seem less important'. This suggests that the value of a *real* baby born through *real* pregnancy overshadows the value of a baby born through surrogacy.

As it emerges in the texts' narratives in focus here, Kate in *Baby Mama* falls pregnant naturally after discovering the surrogate isn't carrying her genetic child. Audrey in *Rules of Engagement* is delighted to acquire her genetic child delivered by her surrogate, but the story concludes with her falling pregnant naturally—the desired happy ending. Charlie accurately described this moment: 'At the end it's like ta dah! You can get pregnant anyway'. The genetic connection, therefore, is not enough, which points to the belief that natural motherhood is a woman's ultimate fulfilment, as 'the core of normal, healthy feminine identity' (Gillespie 2003, 225). Unless they become natural mothers, they misfit—they *fail*.

Much like the 'woman' category in relation to motherhood, it has been proposed through a range of feminist and queer literature that the lesbian has also been viewed as not a *real* woman through the lens of dominant culture, but is, instead, the figure of the *failure* to become a real woman. As Monique Wittig (1992) argued:

> For what makes a woman is a specific social relation to a man, a relation we have previously called servitude, a relation which implies personal and physical obligation as well as economic obligation ("forced residence", domestic corvée, conjugal duties, unlimited production of children, etc.), a relation lesbians escape by refusing to become or stay heterosexual. (1992, 20)

Like the infertile reproductive misfit, the lesbian also misfits—often portrayed as non-normative by not adhering to conventional feminine ideals, as discussed in the previous chapter. As identified by participants Carrie, Jackie, Carla, Sonja and Tara (non-mothers and mixed mothers focus groups), the lesbian—in this discussion, Brenda in *Rules of Engagement*, and the butch couple with a baby in *The New Normal*—are depicted as either overtly masculine with short hair, no make-up dressed in what is culturally perceived as traditional men's clothing, or with unemotional masculine traits which are transformed through pregnancy.

The lesbian has been marginalised through what Rich (1980) has described as a compulsory heterosexuality, a force disseminated through cultural propaganda (magazines, film, literature) that socialises women into the institution of marriage. Rich argues that *only* under this institution of heterosexuality are men and women recognised as *real*. Therefore, I propose that the representations of the characters coping with infertility in these texts share similarities with the lesbian subject position, due to how they have been situated on the outside of social norms. Furthermore, I suggest that this marginalisation also highlights an oppression—and failure—of women (and men) of *other* categories. As Lauren Berlant (2008) identifies, failure is associated with gays, lesbians and those who are, 'unhinged or unhitched, who live outside normative loops of property and reproduction' (2008, 172). Therefore, it is possible to propose that the cultural articulations of infertility in these texts are constructed through the notion that like the lesbian, the infertile woman also disrupts the concept of the normative category 'woman' at its very core and is also excluded.

It is worth mentioning at this juncture, as seen in the work of Cheshire Calhoun (2000), and which has been discussed in Chapter 5 in relation to Brenda's pregnancy in *Rules of Engagement*, that lesbianism and motherhood are seen as incompatible, culturally. Calhoun proposes that lesbian motherhood closets the lesbian subject through the social assumption that motherhood is located purely in the domain of heterosexuality. However, it is important to emphasise at this point that single childless heterosexual women, as illustrated by Kate in *Baby Mama*, share the *other* category of the reproductive technologies' user outside of the white, married, heterosexual couple who dominate popular narratives of infertility. According to Dion Farquhar (1996), these 'Other Mothers' (1996, 73) also include lesbians, those with disabilities, homosexuals and women of colour.

Calhoun argues motherhood masks the subject's lesbianism, as a form of refuge. Therefore, by deflecting the lesbian charge through motherhood, the lesbian subject is brought closer to the category 'woman', and becomes more accepted, tolerated, by heterosexual communities (Calhoun 2000; Lewin 1993; Polikoff 1990). Hence, it has been argued within lesbian activism that refusing to have children, or to give up custody of children during a divorce/separation, is a political manoeuvre by which to refuse participation in compulsory motherhood, the aim being to destabilise the myth of women's fulfilment through motherhood (Burke 1993; Calhoun 2000; Feasey 2017; Klepfisz 1999; Lehr 1999). However, in contrast, some lesbian feminists promote lesbian motherhood, for equality and inclusion, as a form of resistance to the nuclear family kinship model, to allow the natural desires traditionally permitted to heterosexual women (Benkov 1994; Lehr 1999). Arguably this is a result of lesbian motherhood being depicted as non-normative, lesbians seen as unfit for motherhood (Allison 1996; Sourbut 1996; Throsby 2004).[2] The debate on lesbian motherhood is complex, and divisive within lesbian feminism, and has a more nuanced treatment elsewhere (Calhoun 2000; Card 1995; Griffin and Mulholland 1997; Lehr 1999; Lewin 1993; Park 2014; Weston 1991).

Judith Halberstam (2011) identifies in her work on queerness and failure that there are only winners or losers within the conventions of dominant heterosexual society—homosexuals and lesbians only becoming winners by assimilating into dominant culture through obedience to hetero-norms, such as marriage and family. In her work on the narratives of IVF in news stories, Sarah Franklin (1990) has also recognised the winner/loser binary. As also explored in Chapter 2, Franklin argues these stories are constructed around those who get the baby through IVF, and those who don't. Franklin identified in her analysis that the infertile couple stories only find a resolution within the norms of heterosexual marriage. Therefore, the transition from loser to winner (infertile to fertile) through the final equilibrium of natural pregnancy that is constructed in the narratives of both texts is key to this analysis. I argue that this is enabled through the love plot and the formation of the monogamous couple dyad, to be explored further on.

It can be suggested, therefore, that the representations of characters shaped by infertility are creating a clear divide between 'those who breed and those who do not' (O'Brien 1983, 193), which further demonstrates how voids between women are shaped through culture (Sandelowski 1990).[3]

As will be expanded upon, Eve Kosofsky Sedgwick (2008) has argued that Western culture has been structured around the heterosexual/homosexual definition, which is both universalising and minoritising, which she proposes has shaped cultural discourse through the imbalance of power. It is also the rigidity of this binary that implies what is inside or outside power structures, what is seen as natural and unnatural (Fuss 2013). The fertile/infertile binary performs similarly, to both universalise and minoritise, fertility viewed as natural, and infertility as unnatural[4]—much like the deviancy of same-sex desire and coupling and the possibility of building families outside of the heteronormative family unit.

Furthermore, despite the feminisation of the lesbian character in *Rules of Engagement* through pregnancy, as discussed in the previous chapter, and the narrative conclusions of natural pregnancy in both *Rules of Engagement* and *Baby Mama*, the portrayal of the infertile character's relationship to the surrogacy process demonstrates how reproductive technologies have 'altered human's understanding to nature, with paradoxical consequences, especially for women (Lam 2015, 118). Although temporary in both cases, constructed as the disruptions in the narratives, it can be argued that these articulations destabilise the nature/culture binary by removing the intended mothers from the gestational process.

There's Nothing Queer About It

> They [the intended mothers] must feel the way a father must feel.
> (Paula, non-mothers focus group, 2015)

Paula's response to how the intended mothers are portrayed across all of the texts under analysis resonates with Lam's (2015) discussion of how intended mothers are removed from the reproductive process through the intervention of reproductive technologies, such as egg donation and surrogacy, which, as she claims, allows women to feel like fathers.

Lam describes this as 'a new model of birth appropriation by modelling women's material processes of reproduction on men's' which she argues 'most clearly represents the new masculinization of motherhood' (2015, 33). I propose that this masculinisation drives the surrogacy narrative in *Baby Mama*, which is central to the construction of the protagonist Kate, who has been told she is infertile and wishes to acquire a child through the services of a surrogate. As a result of this, a queer reading will expose what I believe to be deeply embedded heterosexist and misogynist ideologies that are ingrained in the text.

As has been suggested, compulsory heterosexuality is articulated through the narratives and scripts that shape our lives. As Ahmed (2004) outlines in her work on queer feelings, a dominant script is that heterosexual coupling is the ideal, and to deviate from this formation would result in unhappiness. The opening scenes in *Baby Mama* inform us that the character of Kate is unmarried due to pursuing a career. As she reveals in the voiceover: 'I made a choice'. Kate later explains that one day her desire for children just suddenly awoke within her: 'I just woke up one day and I felt like every single baby in the street was staring at me'. This reflects the medical and cultural discourse that proposes that voluntary childlessness is just a temporary phase, which will eventually be grown out of (Bartlett 1994; Campbell 1999; Engwall and Peterson 2013). Drawing on Kelly Oliver's (2012) work on pregnancy and Hollywood film, I propose this articulates social anxieties of the career woman in relation to motherhood, the primary fear being that the woman will choose a career instead of a baby.

Kate goes on numerous first dates searching for a partner, and after no success she turns to adoption, which fails. She then tries sperm donation and IVF, which is unfruitful. Like Audrey in *Rules of Engagement*, Kate is depicted as unhappy. She wants a child, and a partner, and is distraught by not being able to get either. This reflects Ahmed's (2010) work on unhappy queers, where she proposes 'such unhappiness is directed toward those who are not living to the right ideas' (2010, 95–96). As Kate's mother says to her during a family meal: 'Not everyone is as tolerant of your alternative lifestyle as we are'. Kate is depicted as being incomplete as a woman, as she is not only incapable of producing a child naturally but is also single. If, as Ahmed proposes, the horizon is shaped by the heteronormative nuclear family, then it can be suggested that the childless characters in both *Baby Mama* and *Rules of Engagement* are not being permitted to be anything *but* unhappy until they acquire their genetic child, which, in these representations, is only achievable through heterosexual coupledom.

To *not* become a natural mother is to be not whole/real, which, as I have suggested, shares an affinity with the lesbian subject position through the failure to be a real woman. Therefore, characters such as Kate *have* to be positioned as lacking, until they are repositioned in approximation to the happy objects of heterosexual romance and the genetic child; objects that 'accumulate affective value as signs of the good life' as they circulate (Ahmed 2010, 38). I propose that if childless characters were positioned as happy, they would be viewed as what Ahmed describes as a 'feminist killjoy' (2010, 25) who causes a disturbance by *choosing* to move away from the happy objects, finding them unhappy. The lesbian surrogate, Brenda, in *Rules of Engagement*, can be described in this way. As discussed in Chapter 3, Brenda became unhappy by being positioned in the proximity of social norms, such as motherhood and family. During a discussion of pregnancy with the younger women (pre-mothers focus group) after the viewing of the texts, Rhian shared a similar stance by declaring she didn't want, or like, children. The room went silent, and her peers gasped and giggled in shock.

> Rhian: I knew I was going to get that reaction.
> Lulu: Was that difficult to admit?
> Rhian: Well, I always feel that people are going to attack me, so I don't like saying it to people.
> (Lulu and Rhian, pre-mothers focus group, 2015)

This moment illustrates what has been described as the contagion of affect (Gibbs 2001) within atmospheres, where 'bodies can catch feelings as easily as catch fire: affect leaps from one body to another, evoking tenderness, inciting shame, igniting rage, exciting fear' (in Gorton 2009, 60). In this moment, Rhian's peers caught the feeling of disgust, which altered the room's atmosphere to one of discomfort. However, this transmission of affect didn't last. After a few moments, Candice quietly explained that their reaction wasn't an attack, and admitted that she had friends who had shared similar feelings. What is evident here is what psychologist and affect theory forerunner Silvan Tomkins (1992) described as the impact of humiliation theory, where the subject in a public space becomes paranoid to negative affect (such as disgust)—anticipating reactions before they happen. As Rhian expressed after the room's atmosphere quickly altered: 'I knew I was going to get that reaction'. Through the negative reaction to her disclosure, Rhian exposes what she infers is her failure to conform to the feminine ideal of being a mother, or more of *wanting* to be a mother which infers she is 'failing to comply' (Edelman 2004, 17) to hetero-norms. This illustrates how childless women are viewed, with 'doubt, suspicion and even disgust' (Engwall and Peterson 2013, 377). This response was evident in the reaction of her peers, even if for just a few moments.

Although Kate in *Baby Mama wants* to be a mother, she is still positioned as non-normative. After a medical examination, Kate's doctor informs her that she has a 'one in a million chance' of getting pregnant. This characterisation and narrative structure reflect Franklin's (1990) claim that in the discourses of infertility in news stories, the medical expert is constructed as key in the movement in the narrative from conflict to resolution, as the only hope. Franklin also identifies how this resolution only emerges in the context of heterosexual union, specifically marriage, which chimes with the proposition that what we think are new stories, such as the narratives of surrogacy in *Baby Mama* and *Rules of Engagement*, are in fact simply repeating conventional notions of family values and women's role in reproduction (Moritz 1987, 1999; Oliver 2012). As explained by Moritz: 'Like history, Hollywood has a way of repeating itself' (1999, 317).

As a single and childless woman, Kate does not fit into the impressions of ideal coupledom carved out by compulsory heterosexuality (Ahmed 2004; Rich 1980). Kate's character could even be described as perverse as she is contesting heteronormative assumptions by opposing 'what is expected, or accepted' (Merck 1993 in Ahmed 2004, 78). Therefore, it can be argued that the narrative is implying that a woman who is single *and* infertile is to be located even further outside dominant social norms, unfit to parent and unable to comply to norms[5] (Edelman 2004; Edge 2014), which further expresses what I have named a *straight queerness*. Kate exhibits all the stereotypical traits of a professional woman going through baby hunger (Hewlett 2002)—a woman who has put her relationships and motherhood on hold in the pursuit of a career, the result being dwindling fertility and a desperation to have a child, through any means possible.

Kate's character draws heavily on the spinster stereotype. The spinster was originally an honourable term used to describe women who spun yarn, its meaning changing in the 1600s to describe an unmarried woman. Its meaning then took on a far more negative connotation in the mid-eighteenth century, when marriage became more idealised socially and culturally, in the reflection of 'the new reverence accorded to wives' (Coontz 2005, 147). The spinster has been prominent in film and TV, commonly represented as single, overweight, frumpy and emotionally unstable (Mustard 2000; Rosenthal 2002). Key examples include contemporary version Bridget in *Bridget Jones Diary* (2001) (big knickers, failed romantic, socially awkward, emotionally unstable) and the more traditional stereotype Charlotte in *Now, Voyager* (1942) (drab, insecure, overweight). Despite being created almost six decades apart, Bridget and Charlotte both transform for the sole purpose to win the love of a good man. Lesbian connotations have also been linked to the spinster stereotype (Jeffreys 1986; McKenna 2002). I argue that Kate, who is emblematic of the new spinster, is perpetuating this stereotype within a similar narrative.

For context, the narrative in *Baby Mama* unfolds like this: the goal (get the baby), equilibrium (engage the surrogate, surrogate gets pregnant), disruption (surrogate is pregnant with her own baby, not Kate's, the two women fall out), resolution (Kate falls in love, gets pregnant), final equilibrium (Kate and the surrogate are best friends again, both have their own babies). During the initial equilibrium stage, the surrogate, Angie, moves in with Kate after she splits from her boyfriend, who, it later transpires, is the father of her baby. The two women bond and Angie, in an attempt to feminise Kate before a girls' night out—the aim being to meet a man—dresses her in what is a culturally marked sexually alluring outfit: a clingy low-cut short dress and high heels. Kate abandons her glasses and is heavily made up. This echoes the spinster transformation moment that reinforces traditional feminine ideals. Kate's romance with the love interest, Rob, sparks at this point when she shows up at his workplace, tipsy. The pair start dating, and she eventually wins the man and later becomes pregnant naturally—lucking out with her one chance out of a million. Kate transforms into a more feminine ideal, 'dressing for male titillation' (Rich 1980, 639), her new appearance also adopting MILF-like (Mother I'd Like to Fuck) qualities, despite not being a mother. However, as May Friedman (2014) has highlighted, the MILF's connection with motherhood is fairly recent, having initially inferred being sexually available, signalled through body-revealing clothes.

Therefore, it is possible to suggest that Kate had to transform into a MILF to become a viable 'maternal subject-in-waiting' (de Benedictis in Littler and Winch 2016, 9) to become eligible for fertility, the pre-mother to the *future foetus* she was searching for. Through this, Kate's newly transformed body has therefore been realigned within the normative; norms of femininity are repeated. This construction, or reshaping, of conventional femininity, through transformation, thereby illustrates what is deemed appropriate desire between men and women (Ahmed 2006; Bartky 1991). She is no longer unfit for potential motherhood as she now qualifies as a good mother through complying to normative gender roles and aspirations of sexuality (Edge 2014; Feasey 2012, 2017; Seidel 2013).

When Kate and surrogate Angie cohabit, it can be proposed that Kate is taking the role as a 'social mother' (Peach 1998). As Deborah Mustard (2000) explains in her work on spinsters in film, women who are not biological mothers often become social mothers 'when they fill a generic mothering role when called upon' (2000, 2). Mustard is referring to spinsters who take care of an elderly parent (*Marvin's Room*, 1996), or an unwanted child (*Baby Boom*, 1987). The surrogate character, Angie, is represented as simple, child-like—she sticks her gum underneath the antique coffee table and is unable to negotiate a baby-proofed apartment. Kate's character can be read a social mother by taking care of Angie like a child. However, in the context of the narrative of family, and the desire for a genetic child, this relationship can be read as sexually ambiguous, as is connoted in how the characters are portrayed and interact. I argue this reveals a heterosexist and misogynistic ideology. As highlighted by Doty (2002), one can't *assume* all film characters are straight unless clearly coded as homosexual or lesbian. Furthermore, through a queer reading, embedded power relations and presumed meanings can be examined and destabilised (Browne and Nash 2010; Gantz 2000). By being single and childless, Kate has fallen off the heterosexual line. Throughout the film, the connotation of a lesbian partnership is conveyed through comedy, in relation to building a family. This resonates with Doty's (1993) analyses of TV shows featuring women living together, which, despite the characters being marked heterosexual, 'hint at the possibility of lesbian lifestyles – at least as far as possible within a dominant ideology' (1993, 44).

Kate and Angie are not the first characters situated in an ambiguous relationship in a popular TV show. Doty (1993) explored the on-screen relationships of the central characters in *Laverne & Shirley* (1976–1983) and *Kate & Allie* (1984–1989). Doty claimed these characters invite a queer reading, often through cases of mistaken identity, or straight characters that 'jokingly play with suggestions of lesbian desire' (1993, 43), all of who, through eventual heterosexual coupling, are able to deflect the lesbian charge. The lesbian connotation in *Baby Mama* follows this. Two women share a domestic space, one of who is pregnant. The narrative infers that the worst thing that can happen in this text is not just to *not* get the baby, but for the women to form an authentic lesbian relationship, or perhaps even worse, end up childless and alone. However, this anxiety was not reflected in the audiences' position on same-sex relationships in relation to building families. As Fay (pre-mothers focus group) stated in response to the differing representations of same-sex coupling across the texts: 'Love is love, it doesn't matter if it's between two women or two men, or a man and a woman. It's natural. It's got nothing to do with gender'.

Following Doty (1993), Rich's concept of the 'lesbian continuum' (1980, 648) is useful to evoke, as the relationship between the two women is not distinctly steered by sexual desire. It appears to be more about the forging of relationships as a potential source of power, 'to embrace many more forms of primary intensity between and among women, including the sharing of a rich inner life, the bonding against male tyranny, the giving and receiving of practical and political support' (Rich 1980, 648–649). This notion of a lesbian continuum emerges at numerous points. These include Kate taking Angie into her home and supporting her through pregnancy (the pregnancy being fake at this point) after her break-up; Kate escorting Angie to the embryo transfer and the antenatal classes; and Kate encouraging Angie to go back to school and be independent, without a man. Angie urges Kate to have more fun in her life.

As noted by Alison Winch (2012) in her analysis of women's films between 2008 and 2009, which she calls 'the girlfriend flick', she claims *Baby Mama* 'attempts to portray the difficulties women face, such as unreliable men, balancing a career, and a desire for motherhood' (2012, 69). Winch further argues these films celebrate supportive friendships with women over romantic relationships. However, Kate and Angie's bonding is illustrated through a pastiche of heterosexual romance, for audience laughs. At their first antenatal class, they are mistaken for a couple. This is shown as a shameful moment by being assumed lesbian (Probyn 2005). Kate and Angie swiftly put the record, and their sexuality, straight. Further in the narrative, after Angie's lie about being pregnant with Kate's foetus has been discovered, the women have an emotional bust-up in a car scene. This provoked an interesting response from Carrie and Sonja (mixed mothers focus group), which was stimulated in the focus group discussion by revisiting the scripted dialogue: 'Angie: You think you're better than me? Kate: Oh, I'm certain I'm better than you'.

> Carrie: Right yes, that was Tina Fey's [Kate] character saying, "I'm certain I'm better than you".
> Sonja: So why did she think she was better than her?
> Carrie: Because she's rich?
> Sonja: Yeah, she was sitting in her car, she was a professional woman, and she had the accoutrements of wealth and success.
> Carrie: And, also Tina Fey's character had sort of, you know, moved her in and invested into the relationship, and was encouraging her to go to college... and this woman was basically trying to fleece her, so I agree, I think she was better than her.
> (Carrie and Sonja, mixed mothers focus group, 2015)

Although the focus group participants weren't reading the characters' relationship directly as lesbian, what did emerge was an acknowledgement of an intense dynamic between the two women, which surfaced through what Christine Geraghty (2003) calls 'emotional explosions' (in Gorton 2009, 75)—a device in the narrative structure that constructs an emotional connection with the viewer. Tension between the women is built further in this scene when Angie turns to Kate and says: 'Okay, we're being honest now? Here's one. I can have a baby and you can't. And that drives you crazy'. This accentuates Sandelowski's (1990) argument that fictional representations of infertile women 'promotes motherhood and subverts sisterhood' (1990, 34) by pitching women against each other by an ability to procreate, naturally.[6]

Carrie and Sonja have identified the power imbalance between the two characters. Kate has money and is successful. Angie has nothing apart from the foetus Kate is willing to pay $100k for. What is revealed in this exchange is one of the genre's key conventions. By Carrie reading that Angie was trying to 'fleece' Kate by lying about the baby for money, she is inferring that betrayal between two women is worse than losing trust in a man (Winch 2012). As seen in the work of Winch, lying about being pregnant, and/or being pregnant by someone else—in this case, Angie's ex-boyfriend—is the ultimate betrayal. This disruption in the narrative borrows from melodrama, which is core to soap opera. This is created through editing, music, camera angles, acting and the sequence of scenes, which portray high emotions, moral opposition, scheming and suspense. Due to its ability to manipulate the viewer in the evocation of emotional response, and its 'lack of aesthetic distance' (Williams 1991, in Gorton 2009, 79), melodrama has been deemed of a lower cultural status, seen primarily as a woman's genre (Gledhill 1987; Neale 2000).

Melodrama, of the more dramatic and less comedic incarnation, emerged in the 1950s through the work of filmmaker Douglas Sirk, and has been traced even further back to sentimental novels of the eighteenth and nineteenth century (Elsaesser 1973; Willemen 1971). This inferior cultural position implies that women's social position is also viewed as lower status, female concerns are seen as having lesser value (Gledhill 1987). I propose this view of women's social position is evident in *Baby Mama*, through how the infertile characters have been constructed within the narrative. This has been illuminated through what has been described as the feminisation of the genre, shaped in relation to discourses of family and motherhood (Brunsdon 1997; Gorton 2009; Moseley 2003). For example, through the rom-com emerged the mom-com, motherhood being the primary goal, ahead of romance.

This can be identified in Fay and Rhian's (pre-mothers focus group) comments in relation to this particular narrative drive:

> Rhian: In *Baby Mama* she didn't have a partner. There was no love at first but she wanted a child *to love*.
>
> Fay: And she was excited when she found out, even though she didn't have a partner.
>
> Lulu: So, the baby brings the love to her?
>
> Rhian: Yeah… It's like, when you get to a certain stage you need a baby, otherwise your life is pointless.
>
> (Rhian, Fay and Lulu, pre-mothers focus group, 2015)

This response demonstrates what I have named the delayed conception plotline. However, although Rhian and Fay are able to recognise this love-desire for a child is the primary goal in the storyline, through what has been earlier described as a baby hunger, both participants are aware that such notions are an expectation, and not what either of them believe in—the notion of completeness through motherhood being a myth perpetuated by popular narratives (Klepfisz 1999). Myths circulating in popular culture and in everyday life of what is required to be fulfilled as a woman are explored further in Chapter 5.

The mom-com, therefore—or in this context what should be more aptly entitled the *pre-mom-com* due to the pursuit of the *future foetus*—evidences the fetishisation of the maternal that has saturated popular culture. As Halberstam (2011) has identified in the happy endings of romantic comedies, the female orgasm has to date been the 'frothy white dresses' and 'over-the-top cakes'—the 'consummation of all the hopes and dreams that young women have been offered along the way to adulthood' (2011, 116). The delayed conception plotline therefore describes the shift from the celebratory conclusion of the wedding, to the celebratory conclusion of the baby. This is symbolic of the inscription of femininity, what it means to be a *real* woman: to be a mother.

Laura Mumford (1995) claims that although the paternal plotline is soap opera's defining characteristic, there is potential for more maternal-centred plots to emerge through the growing popularity of reproductive technologies, as the genre is watched predominantly by women. As Mumford explains:

> Although adoption and adultery have been the soaps' traditional solutions to characters' fertility problems, changes in the social and technological relations of reproduction will no doubt mean changes in fictional "solutions" as well… It is easy to imagine a future maternity plot whose central mystery is whether a pregnancy was the result of an embryo transplant or "normal" conception. (1995, 103)

Baby Mama demonstrates this shift, as the plotline introduces surrogacy as a fertility solution. The melodramatic device of the paternal plotline, therefore, has progressed to a maternal plotline. In the context of this text, this infers a betrayal between the two women. Not who is the daddy, but who is the mummy. In the latter part of the film, the two women go to court to legitimise, through blood tests, which of them is the genetic mother, clarifying whether the pregnancy is the result of, as foreseen by Mumford, an embryo transplant or normal conception. This can be read as infidelity outside of their played-for-laughs relationship, as previously highlighted, while also alluding to the bigger maternal question in relation to the surrogacy as a practice. The legal mother of a baby born from surrogacy differs globally due to inconsistencies in the law.

Due to the ambiguous nature of their relationship, the car scene when Kate drops Angie off at a hotel after their bust-up can be given a queer reading, though how they have been positioned, literally. The object of the car idealises heterosexual romance, an intimate space which has become commonplace in popular cultural representations (Ahmed 2006). It can be suggested that this scene is a break-up scene, a trope frequently employed in romantic comedy, which is followed by a make-up scene (McDonald 2007).

In *Baby Mama*, this emerges in a later scene when the surrogate Angie goes into labour, and Kate is there to support her. In the car scene, an angry and emotional Angie says to Kate: 'So you're done with me now is that it? You don't need me anymore?' It appears Angie is performing the role of the jilted lover. The power dynamic between the two women is being played out through the adoption of masculine and feminine roles. Sonja described Kate as a 'professional woman' who has the 'accoutrements of wealth and success'. Carrie read Kate as superior to Angie, due to 'investing' in the relationship by moving her into her home, and encouraging her to study, which suggests the 'giving of practical support' (Rich 1980, 648). Sonja and Carrie read Kate's traits as masculine through her economic and professional position. These traits are reinforced through how she is seated behind the wheel. As queer media scholar Katherine Gantz (2000) proposes, through her analysis of a car scene featuring two men in hit American sitcom *Seinfeld*, this demonstrates a parody of the heterosexual dating scene, and that being seated behind the wheel is representative of masculine power.

Paula's (non-mothers focus group) statement of: 'They [the intended mothers] must feel the way a father must feel' has further explanatory power here to explore how Kate's masculine characteristics within the narrative have been formed, in relation to, and in relationship with, Angie, her surrogate. Kate and Angie's characters have been developed through the heterosexual dyad of father/mother, masculine/feminine. This is a dualism that has shaped the sitcom formula, which, alongside soap opera, has also influenced film comedy. As has been explored in more depth in the analysis of male same-sex parenting in *The New Normal* and *Modern Family*, as discussed in Chapter 3, hints of the lesbian concept butch–femme also re-emerge here, through the binary division of father/mother into masculine/feminine. This illuminates the masculinisation of Kate's character by her being removed from the conception and birthing process—until she falls pregnant naturally as the final equilibrium.

It is important to emphasise the imbalance of power that is created through the construction of these binary hierarchies, as the rigidity of the boundary is restrictive, as it subordinates one over the other, excludes one over the other (Fuss 2013; Sedgwick 2008). Sedgwick argues that the emergence of the heterosexual/homosexual binary has been hugely influential on the organisation of Western culture, even beyond homosexual identity and culture, socially organising identities and definitions into two category polarities, particularly in relation to gender, class and race, which is poignant in relation to the discussion of the representations of parental roles and gender identity in these texts.

As I have suggested previously, butch–femme as a concept materialises in the characterisation of same-sex couples, to reinforce what is deemed as an acceptable mode of parenting, through the stereotyping of gender roles. Through the representation of both female (although ambiguous) and male same-sex couples explored in this thesis, I further propose that this mimics heterosexual culture rather than subverting it. The masculine/feminine, butch–femme traits/traces also emerge through how the characters are dressed, perform, and their professional and economic status. Before Kate's feminine transformation, her style was masculine, frumpy—a dress code in line with the construction of the spinster stereotype.

Although her character is culturally marked female by having long hair, her look appears more androgynous rather than overtly masculine, which suggests that the character's sexual identity is more ambiguous than clearly coded lesbian. As Brenda Weber (2009) highlights in her work on TV show transformations, the purpose of the makeover is to eradicate any ambiguities, which also includes erasing shame, which as has been argued must be evoked for the makeover transformation to take place (Doyle and Irmgard 2008; Gill 2007; McRobbie 2004; Peck 1995; Skeggs and Wood 2012; Walkerdine 2011). Kate transforms into a woman that will be desired by men (which erases the shame of infertility and spinsterhood) becoming a female body that adheres to the codes of conventional femininity (Bartky 1991; Weber 2009). Towards the end of the film, Angie also transforms (erasing the shame of poverty, class) when she is now situated as an (almost) equal to Kate, as friends, when they are pictured together with their children at Angie's daughter's first birthday party. I return to this scene in the discussion of rescue later in the chapter. Furthermore, what this scene also demonstrates is what Rebecca Feasey (2017) describes as a maternal hierarchy between mother characters who are bad, barely good enough, and just good enough—configurations that build voids between women (Sandelowski 1990). In *Baby Mama*, as the surrogate character, it can be suggested that Angie is 'good enough' as she *chooses* to become a mother to the baby, unlike Brenda in *Rules of Engagement* and Goldie in *The New Normal* who both happily renounce all parental responsibility at the baby's birth. The key difference being that as it transpired Angie was carrying her genetic foetus, and not Kate's, which highlights the value connected to the genetic bond through the ideology of normative reproduction. Love bond and the genetic tie are explored further in the following chapter.

In contrast to Kate's character, Angie has bleach-blonde hair and dresses in a more feminine, but less expensive fashion style. Carrie (mixed mothers focus group) was able to position Angie within the feminine category by describing her character as 'white, virginal and blonde'. Nadra, in the same group, detected similarities between the surrogates in both *Baby Mama* and *The New Normal*, who she described as dumb blondes that 'look just the same'. These descriptions of race and hair colour point towards the value of whiteness in the construction of conventional femininity (Dyer 1993, 1997; Loyo in Everett 2007). Aside from the blonde stereotype in popular cultural representations inferring idiocy, blonde is also a category that marks the subject as white. Interestingly, however, in the case of the two surrogate characters, they are positioned as subordinate to the primary characters, but in relation to fertility which infers femininity. However, whiteness doesn't always denote privilege—the white surrogates in these two texts are also positioned as subordinate through the class divisions that have been constructed between them, shaped by the stereotype of white trash that marks the characters as inferior, as well as the divisive tensions between the fertile and infertile that have been shaped in the narrative (Sandelowski 1990; Tyler 2008).

Susan Berridge and Karen Boyle (2014) argue that it is the class division that has been created between them that obstructs any lesbian possibilities, as it is class that marks them as incompatible. During the baby shower scene in *Baby Mama*, during the melodramatic reveal moment when Kate finds out Angie has been lying about her pregnancy, Kate calls Angie 'ignorant white trash' which is symbolic of class disgust (Tyler 2008). Since *Baby Mama's* release in 2018, the white trashing of female characters on TV has increased, which has been identified as jumping on a white trash bandwagon[7] (Feasey 2017). Charlotte Hayes (2013) claims the construction of these characters can also be interpreted as a form of car crash TV for audience pleasure. However, in this study, the participants in the focus groups did not express pleasure. They were appalled at the white trash statement, as Tara (non-mothers focus group) explained: 'I was really shocked when there was this whole thing of, you know, "ignorant white trash", and you know, low life… that was their [*Baby Mama's*] running theme of socio-economic hierarchy of who carries a child and who pays for that person. That was really prominent'. Angie's character embodies the white trash stereotype not just through the character's poverty inferred by the surrogacy arrangement, but through the cheapness of her clothes, lack of education, dishonesty and ignorance of foetal neglect through nutrition, as discussed in the previous chapter. For example, both Angie in *Baby Mama* and Goldie in *The New Normal* eat junk food, which the intended parents attempt to rectify. This reflects how the stereotype of white trash demonstrates an appropriation of racist American political rhetoric which views blacks as a failing underclass who neglect their foetuses. In addition, this stereotype also demonstrates how negative images of working-class motherhood continue to dominant popular culture as a method of marginalisation, depicting them as 'ignorant, promiscuous, uncaring, irresponsible and most significantly, undeserving' (Gillies 2006 in Feasey 2015, 26).

Race and infertility are significant in the discussion of these texts. As emphasised by scholars in the field of race and reproductive technologies, the medical and media discourse of infertility is constructed as white, heterosexual, married and middle class (Franklin 1990; Hewlett 2002; Roberts 1996). In the context of this chapter, the constructions of the childless characters Kate in *Baby Mama* and Audrey in *Rules of Engagement*, imply that reproductive technologies are only accessible to the white, middle classes, bodies that are *permitted* and supported to transform—to be rescued—to reproduce racially pure children of the future (Roberts 1996).

It is imperative to mention how the black characters in these texts are positioned to enable the future happiness of the white characters. Drawing on Berlant (2008) I propose this characterisation within the narrative idealises white sentimentality. In *Baby Mama*, Oscar, the black doorman, supports the lead white characters by providing committed, emotional support. He was the first to discover the surrogate Angie was lying about the pregnancy, encouraging her to do the right thing and come clean. As Carrie (mixed mothers focus group) stated in response to the character: 'Doormen are always wise, aren't they?'

The character of Rocky in *The New Normal* also plays a supportive role. As the lead character's personal assistant and best friend, Bryan's needs are placed ahead of hers, which infers subordination through ideologies of both race *and* gender. Following the depiction of black characters of the 1970–1980s, both of these black characters are shown as not only of lower-class status 'but with lower educational and occupational status' (Sweeper 1984).[8]

I propose these representations are constructed through heterosexist, sexist, and racist ideologies that emerge through conventional notions of family values, fit parenthood, whiteness, femininity, and women's role in reproduction. The character of Kate, in particular, has been situated in opposition to the patriarchal status quo, by being depicted as single and experiencing infertility, which, as has been argued, positions her as non-normative. As Oliver (2012) argues, for a woman in a film storyline to have a career, but not the baby, is the worst thing that can happen.

Someday My Prince Will Come

> The worst thing is not to get the baby, or not to have a baby. That doesn't happen there, in that world, because there's always a way, and that's really weird, that's really weird as it's creating this kind of stick we're supposed to be beating ourselves with.
>
> (Carla, mixed mothers focus group, 2015)

Oliver's evaluation of how an independent professional woman is positioned in the narrative as devalued, unless she has a child, can be clearly identified in Carla's statement. As Carla describes, the worst outcome possible is to not get the baby, which materialises in the disruption moment in the narrative structure, when Kate discovers that her surrogate Angie has lied about carrying her genetic foetus. Through Carla's description of 'that world', what can be recognised, drawing on Berlant (2008), is a constructed and mediated fantasy of the normative. Through this fantasy world, as Carla has identified, 'there's always a way'. The final equilibrium in the narrative is when Kate falls pregnant naturally, and acquires the *real* baby she desired, enabled through the device of the heterosexual love plot. This unfolding of the narrative therefore relocates the infertile character from a non-normative position to a normative one. This highlights further that heterosexual women have more reproductive options than lesbians. As previously mentioned in relation to groupings of persons who use technologies for reproductive freedom, heterosexual women *can* utilise procedures such as IVF and surrogacy, whereas lesbians *must*—it is their *only* choice.

Berlant claims that sentimentality shapes the ideology of heterosexual love through textual intervention, that it is circular as it drives the repetitive motion of heterosexual love through the stories that are told, with their promises of redemption. In the context of this discussion, this is reflected in the transition from infertile to fertile, lesbian ambiguity to heterosexual clarity, non-normative to normative—outside to inside. This narrative pattern has been detected in all of the texts under analysis and will be explored further in Chapter 5. This repetition of impressions, as seen in the work of Ahmed (2006), allows the *right type* of bodies (white, middle class, heterosexual) to 'extend into spaces that have already taken their shape' (2006, 425). These are spaces that have been shaped by compulsory heterosexuality. Berlant argues that women's culture in America, specifically, markets particular notions of femininity to female audiences, which aims to 'span fantasy and experience and claim a certain emotionality amongst women' (2008, 5). This ideology of the normative, in this analysis, is that to be feminine is to be heterosexual *and* to be a natural mother, which is enabled through the love of a man. As Irena Klepfisz (1999) describes in relation to her own experiences, childless women—particularly those who don't marry—are stigmatised, characterised as cold, unfeminine, unnatural. This is an accurate description of Kate's character, pre-transformation and positioned as sexually ambiguous. Furthermore, this description also illustrates the tropes of women in popular representations who have *rejected* motherhood, particularly within the thriller and horror genres. Drawing on film noir's femme fatale (Grossman 2009; Hanson 2007; Cook 1998), this character of the childfree *monstrous* woman is presented as emotionally unstable and dangerous—Catherine in *Basic Instinct* (1992) (who kills her lover with an ice pick during sex), Hedy in *Single White Female* (1992) (who kills her roommate's husband by gauging out his eye with a stiletto heel) and Alex in *Fatal Attraction* (1987) (who kills her ex-lover's family's pet rabbit and self-harms). Hedy in *Single White Female*, who displays lesbian tendencies, is killed off as the narrative's final resolution. This reflects the common killing off of lesbian characters in popular culture, as touched upon in Chapter 5. As seen in the work of Edelman (2004) and Oliver (2012), this choice to non-procreate signifies a bleakly populated future—the undoing of life itself. The childless woman as a reproductive threat is explored in the following chapter. Popular representations infer, then, that a woman who chooses *not* to have children is deficient and non-normative. Therefore, I believe that the narrative in *Baby Mama* aims to reinforce the value of conventional normative femininity and heterosexuality, that women are better placed in heterosexual partnerships, placing moral importance on the building of family through natural procreation.

As discussed, the narrative in *Baby Mama* plays with the lesbian joke. Kate is single and wants a baby. The disruption in the story is the possibility of *not* getting the baby, which is resolved through Kate becoming pregnant naturally through the love of a man. As Berlant (2008) has argued, the heterosexual love plot is motivated by the desire for normativity, where narratives invest in specific ideas of femininity—in this analysis, notions of fertility, heterosexuality and whiteness. Berlant's concept of the blockage, in relation to the love plot, is useful to mobilise here to examine this disruption stage, primarily to explore how both lesbianism *and* infertility are rendered invisible in the narrative. The blockage is central to the genre's successful execution, as it conjures the prospect of failure. It is the threat that 'x might *not* happen… which allows absorbing but not shocking anxieties to be stimulated and vanquished' (Berlant 2008, 19). This disruption, or threat of failure, is an integral narrative device, as the resolution and final equilibrium follow, to overcome anxieties and enable the heteronormative happy ending. In *Baby Mama*, as emphasised by Carla, the 'x' is to 'not get the baby', which I argue symbolises the failure to become a *real* woman. However, Carla was unable to recognise that alongside not getting the baby, the worst thing that could also happen is to become a lesbian or remain single. I propose that the lesbian charge has been submerged through the love plot, which, as argued by Winch (2012), steers the narrative to the resolution stage, 'where heterosexual men provide relief from the scrutinizing gaze' (2012, 77).

Although Kate's character is not lesbian-identified, her masculine traits and infertility situate her within this blockage in the narrative, which Berlant also describes as an 'interruption', which is when the subject's—or in this discussion, character's—world is fragile and vulnerable, the fantasy of the good life placed out of reach. Through Kate's characterisation, she is displaying, drawing on Berlant, a 'feminine fraying' (2008, 18) when femininity becomes undone, and heterosexuality is in crisis. I argue that this fraying provides the tension point in the blockage/disruption in the narrative of *Baby Mama*, which I propose appears in the ambiguous relationship between Kate and Angie. The love plot and the makeover, as previously discussed, rescue the characters and erase all ambiguities, Kate being repositioned as feminine through her desire to be a mother, and her longing to be sexually attractive to a man. Her femininity has been reorientated on the straight line. She is now facing the right way towards heterosexual happiness (Ahmed 2006, 2010). Kate has transformed from loser to winner, through the shift from infertile to fertile—the stigma disappears. Kate has corrected her failing by not resisting the constraints of compulsory heterosexuality that, as pinpointed by Cohen (1997), can be viewed as a system of dominance that seeks to 'normalize our sexuality, exploit our labour, and constrain our visibility' (1997, 440)—acting as a blockage to the lesbian possibility (Ahmed 2006; Rich 1980).

What has been represented as non-normative (masculine traits, single, childless, two women living together, surrogacy) has transformed into the normative (heterosexual pairing/love, natural pregnancy, femininity) which is, as Berlant proposes, the utopian dream as marketed through women's popular cultural texts. In these texts, the couple is the central focus and is core to normative love (Ahmed 2006; Berlant 2008). Through Kate's transformation in the narrative, the monogamous heterosexual couple is deemed as legitimate, performing the work to maintain hierarchy within the institution of heterosexuality (Ahmed 2010; Berlant 2008; Berlant and Warner 1998; Duggan 2002; Foucault 1998).

In addition, in the context of *Baby Mama's* central surrogacy storyline, the insertion of the heterosexual couple in relation to romantic love and reproduction is also a vehicle for placating anxieties surrounding new reproductive technologies—primarily the creation of babies through non-coital methods. As Oliver (2012) identifies: 'While we are used to seeing sex without love in contemporary Hollywood films, we are not used to seeing babies without sex… Uncoupling sex and reproduction causes so much anxiety that, often in the most contrived ways, these films manage to bring them back together' (2012, 69). This statement also highlights further anxieties in relation to female sexuality, as through this 'uncoupling' what also emerges is the threat of the lesbian possibility, a threat *to* heterosexuality and to normative womanhood, all of which *must* be submerged in the narrative in the central pursuit of natural, genetic reproduction, which is evident, if not over-determined, in all of the texts discussed in this book.

Berlant claims that the love plot acts as a form of disappointment management for female audiences through the cultivation of fantasies. This, she argues, enables women to belong to a larger world, to experience love affectively as a form of diversion. This resonates with Janice Radway's (1983, 1992) work on the female readers of romance novels, where she argued, through her audience data, that the fantasy of romance allowed the reader to escape from their everyday lives. As Berlant argues, which echoes this, it's the fictional love plot that 'transports people somewhere into a *situation* for a minute' (Berlant 2008, 31). This notion of transportation further reflects Gorton's (2009) earlier proposition that audiences wish to *feel* something through how they connect with and relate to the narrative, and to experience the emotions the characters are portrayed as feeling, particularly through the episodic flow of sitcoms and soap operas. As Gorton explains: 'A text's ability to move us emotionally is not simply an aesthetic value but also a political one. The presence of emotion in popular television move its viewers to feel a sense of connectedness and belonging that is repeated in each episode' (2009, 78). Although the two texts under discussion are a film and a sitcom, the strategies are akin to how women are portrayed on primetime American television, in relation to methods of production and modes of representation (Kuhn 1992; Moritz 1987, 1999).

The fantasy in *Baby Mama* and *Rules of Engagement* is that women's infertility can be magically cured through heterosexual love. Not only does love rescue Kate from her life as a single, childless woman, but it also saves her from the lesbian possibility. As Berlant highlights: 'The modern love plot requires that, if you are a woman, you must at least *entertain* believing in love's capacity both to rescue you from your life and to give you a new one' (2008, 171). In this analysis, the love plot and the couple dyad has enabled Kate (*Baby Mama*) and Audrey (*Rules of Engagement*) to become natural mothers. They have been able to shed their old bodies and claim better, fertile ones, transforming them into the conventional feminine ideal.

Through this notion of rescue, it can be argued that the love plot in *Baby Mama* is a contemporary reworking of the classic fairy tale narrative that drives most love stories. Kathleen Barry (1985), Valerie Walkerdine (1984), and Rich (1980) have argued that the fairy tale narrative presents a version of heterosexual romance to pre-adolescent girls as a form of social conditioning. This, they claim, acts as a form of indoctrination that beams out of comics, TV, advertising, films and songs. Walkerdine argues that comics in particular offer a happy ever after situation in which 'the finding of the prince (the knight in shining armour, 'Mr. Right') comes to seem like a solution to a set of overwhelming desires and problems' (in McRobbie and Nava 1984, 163). In these tales, Walkerdine proposes that getting the man (the prince) is the final solution. I propose that the narrative in *Baby Mama* is doing the same thing. The beautiful girl (Kate, post-makeover) gets a reward for her good deeds (trying to help the surrogate) and is eventually taken out of her misery and is freed by the prince (Kate's love interest Rob rescues her from a life of lesbianism and childlessness). Therefore, this implies that the heterosexual line is only stable if female bodies are constructed for men. As Ahmed (2006) argues, such bodies point *towards* men, and are occupied by men (penetration).

Through the device of the rescue narrative, Kate's career path has also been thwarted. She is shown at the end of the film at Angie's daughter's first birthday party, surrounded by the kinship objects (Ahmed 2006) of children's toys, party food and balloons, seated in a children's play area. Drawing on Ahmed (2010), this scene displays a 'ground of happiness', where the 'happy folk' are—Kate finally has 'what they have' (2010, 112). This is the antithesis of how her character was introduced at the film's beginning. Through the impact of heterosexual coupling and pregnancy, Kate's character has not only been straightened, she has been domesticated. Through her lesbian ambiguity and infertility being cured through the love of a man, she has been restored to her proper place within the traditional family structure, a common narrative resolution in cinema, as a form of restoration (Cook 1998; Kuhn 1992; Moritz 1999; Walker 1982). Annette Kuhn (1992) explains that this is executed in several ways: 'a woman character may be restored to the family by falling in love, by "getting her man", by "getting married", or otherwise accepting a "normative" female role' (in Moritz 1999, 317).[9] This reflects conventional ideas of domesticity which Estella Tinckell (2005) claims emerged in popular culture as a response to the sharp rise in married women in the workplace post the Second World War. Tinckell explores this through her reading of career-girl-turns-mother movies *Pillow Talk* (1959) and *Lover Come Back* (1962). She claims these films imply that women choosing work over motherhood is a form of resistance which takes the love of a man to remind her of her proper position—in the home.[10] *Baby Mama* repeats the same narrative.

However, the final resolution is not just about being rescued by the prince, but is, in addition, about being rescued through the normalisation of natural conception, which has been enabled through the love interest character (Rob, *Baby Mama*) or a stable male partner (Jeff, *Rules of Engagement*). In *Rules of Engagement*, as has been previously discussed, despite Audrey and Jeff acquiring a genetic child through surrogacy, it is not the American dream of a conventional family. Therefore, the final equilibrium is when Audrey faints during the surrogate's labour, and discovers she is pregnant—a scene also mirrored in *Baby Mama*. The difference being Kate's surrogate was birthing her own genetic child, and not Kate's. As identified by Sonja (mixed mothers focus group):

> Maybe it's not a happy ending, maybe it's not good enough that the surrogate mother has given birth to a child for you, maybe that's not good enough, maybe that's not the fairytale.
>
> (Sonja, mixed mothers focus group, 2015)

What can be identified in Sonja's statement is how the fairy tale narrative is integral to the construction of the texts' narratives, specifically in relation to the social and cultural value of normative reproduction that materialises in *Rules of Engagement*. Laura (non-mothers focus group) also pinpoints, like Sonja, how the text suggests that to have a child through surrogacy is not enough:

> It's not necessarily a sad ending if they can't have children, because we knew that from the beginning that they couldn't. If they have a child through surrogacy, they've got a child. It doesn't mean they have to get pregnant by natural means to conclude the story, to complete her as a person and as a woman.
>
> (Laura, non-mothers focus group, 2015)

Like Sonja, Laura is pointing to a shift in the narrative, through the affective value attached to the arrival of a baby procured 'by natural means'. She argues that the narrative 'concludes the story' by completing the characters through this transformational process. By rejecting the dominant codes embedded in the narrative, what can be revealed is how audiences (in this sample) believe that such an ending should not be wholly representative of a feminine desire for normative reproduction. Through both Laura and Sonja's responses, what can be acknowledged is that heterosexual love and natural motherhood are being depicted as essential to normative femininity (Berlant 2008). Kate in *Baby Mama* has transformed to not just get the man, but the baby, too—her primary desire. There has been a narrative shift. It is no longer about 'the moment of bliss that is signified by the first kiss' (Walkerdine in McRobbie and Nava 1984, 176). The final resolution in these texts is not the arrival of the prince after all, but the arrival of the baby.

However, Carla (mixed mothers focus group) takes a position that is oppositional to Berlant's claim that the cultivation of fantasies through women's texts creates feelings of belonging. As described in the introduction of this section, Carla highlights how the fantasy of the heterosexual love plot 'in that world' creates 'this kind of stick we are supposed to be beating ourselves with'. Rather than finding comfort through the affective device of sentimentality and the cultivation of fantasy, she finds discomfort. She *doesn't* belong. The narrative is encoded with the ideology of fulfilment, that to become a natural mother is to become *whole*. Carla's response indicates that her discomfort places her *outside* of belonging, contrary to Berlant's argument that the love plot offers a point of identification that can enable a sense of fitting in. Berlant emphasises the sense of belonging that is constructed through mass-mediated culture only relates to those who are already situated as conventional.

In the discussion of how characters diagnosed with infertility are portrayed in these texts, culturally shaped notions and expectations of what is deemed normative and non-normative in the context of womanhood, motherhood, family and femininity have been presented. Specifically, how a woman must be characterised to fit in, through 'accepting a "normative" female role' (Kuhn 1992 in Moritz 1999, 317). Through textual analysis and audience work, a number of core ideologies have been identified: completeness, natural reproduction, romance, heterosexuality and whiteness. However, what has emerged as significant through the audience analysis is how the participants have mostly rejected the dominant narratives of family and motherhood in both *Baby Mama* and *Rules of Engagement*. As Laura stated: 'It's not necessarily a sad ending if they can't have children'. Therefore, a discussion of the participants' resistance to the texts, while also recognising their astute reflexivity to the genre mechanisms and a desire to see alternative happy endings, will be explored in the following chapter.

Notes

1. In her discussion Cohen (1997) was referring to the intersection of race and heterosexuality, and the exclusion of black heterosexual bodies from dominant white heterosexual culture. However, in the context of this chapter her argument against the monolithicity of heterosexuality is still relevant. In addition, her racial perspective on heterosexuality is also useful to consider when exploring the construction of the infertile bodies in the texts as white, coupled and middle class.
2. The hetero-turned lesbian adoptive mother character Julia (played by Nicole Kidman) in *Top of the Lake: China Girl* is depicted as incompatible with motherhood as her 18-year-old adopted daughter Mary shows nothing but contempt for her lesbian identity, preferring to embrace a new bond with her heterosexual birth mother, Robin (played by Elisabeth Moss). It can be argued here that by becoming a lesbian Julia disrupted the category 'woman', hence positioning her as non-normative and therefore excluded from the family centre. As (assumed) infertile *and* a lesbian this is a double disruption, much like Kate in *Baby Mama*—where a lesbian relationship is inferred for audience laughs. The character of Julia is constructed as unstable emotionally and love-sick for her estranged daughter. Julia's relationship with her lesbian partner falters. The final resolution in the narrative is when Mary returns to a happier stable home—her adopted parents are reunited, the nuclear family model restored. This illustrates how heterosexual love rescues the deviant lesbian—she is redeemed and repositioned back on the heterosexual straight line (Ahmed 2010). The heterosexual love plot is discussed in Chapter 5, and *Top of the Lake: China Girl* is discussed further in Chapter 6.
3. Pitting women against each other for commercial entertainment can be identified across a wide range of popular media content. Examples include Meghan Markle vs Kate Middleton, Diana Spencer vs Sarah Ferguson, Angelina Jolie vs Jennifer Aniston. Sarah Ferguson's open letter published in *Hello* magazine in February 2019 called out the media's tactics of pitting women against each other to sell newspapers. This unsisterly technique has also provided narrative fuel for TV and film programming, seen in reality TV shows such as *Wife Swap* (Channel 4 2003–2009), *The Real Housewives of...* series, and movies such as *Mean Girls* (2004) and *Bride Wars* (2009). Muller, "Calls Out Media".
4. LGTBQ communities can also be included here due to being neglected from cultural narratives of infertility (Walks 2007).
5. The lead character Robin in *Top of the Lake: China Girl* is also portrayed as unfit for motherhood. It can be argued in the context of this debate that this is due to her deviancy as a single woman who not only chooses a career over domesticity, but that her biological daughter Mary was

the result of a gang rape when she was a teenager, whom she put up for adoption.

6. This is a key narrative device that continues to emerge for TV entertainment, particularly in programmes with surrogacy storylines. In TV dramas *Top of the Lake: China Girl* and *The Handmaid's Tale*, this tension between the fertile and infertile female characters are at the centre of the narratives. The complexities of these relationships in the context of the drama genre is discussed in Chapter 6.
7. Shows that demonstrate this white trash bandwagon include *Mom* (CBS 2013–present), *Here Comes Honey Boo Boo* (TLC 2012–2017) which followed on from shows such as *Shameless* (Channel 4 2004–2013) and *Ladette to Lady* (ITV 2005–2008) (see Feasey 2017; Hayes 2013).
8. The support of white sentimentality can also be identified in the construction of the Thai surrogates in *Top of the Lake: China Girl*. All of the intended parents in the story are white. The women of colour are contracted to produce white babies to enable their future happiness. In this case, however, the Thai surrogates return home with the intended parents' precious cargo in utero, leaving the couples distraught. This dramatic exit was staged as a political act—for the intended parents there was no happy ending. This is discussed in Chapter 6.
9. This narrative is also evident in *Baby Boom* (1987) where highflying management consultant J. C. Wiatt (even her name is masculinised) who has no time for romance, suddenly inherits an estranged relative's small child. She leaves her career to look after the child, moves out of the city, sets up a gourmet baby food business and falls in love.
10. An exaggerated example of this is illustrated in *The Handmaid's Tale* where traditional gender roles for women are compulsory by law. Women and girls are not allowed to read, be educated or work. Aside from the handmaids being forced to reproduce against their will, the structure of the household also replicates the patriarchal home of the seventeenth century. The wife forced to chastity, the husband free sexually. The wife's only role being the head servant of the household. As explained by Frederick Engels: 'The man seized the reigns also in the house, the women were stripped of their dignity, enslaved, tools of men's lust and mere machines for the generation of children' (2001, 70).

References

Ahmed, Sara. 2004. *The Cultural Politics of Emotion*. London: Routledge.

Ahmed, Sara. 2006. *Queer Phenomenology: Orientations, Objects, Others*. London: Routledge.

Ahmed, Sara. 2010. *The Promise of Happiness*. Durham: Duke University Press.

Alcoff, Linda. 2006. *Race, Gender, and the Self.* New York: Oxford University Press.
Allison, Christine. 1996. "The Making of a Bad Mother: A Lesbian Mother and Her Daughters." In *Between Monsters, Goddesses and Cyborgs: Feminist Confrontations with Science, Medicine and Cyberspace*, edited by Nina Lykke and Rosi Braidotti. London: Zed Books.
Ally McBeal. 1997–2002. Created by Dave E. Kelley. TV programme. Los Angeles, CA: Fox.
Ashurst, Pamela, and Zaida Hall. 1989. *Understanding Women in Distress.* London: Routledge.
Baby Mama. 2008. Directed and written by Michael McCullers. Film. Universal City, CA: Universal Pictures.
Barry, Kathleen. 1985. *Female Sexual Slavery.* New York: New York University Press.
Bartky, Sandra. 1991. *Femininity and Domination: Studies in the Phenomenology of Oppression.* London: Routledge.
Bartlett, Jane. 1994. *Will You Be a Mother Who Chooses to Say No?* London: Virago.
Benkov, Laura. 1994. *Reinventing the Family: The Emerging Story of Lesbian and Gay Parents.* New York: Crown Publishers.
Berlant, Lauren. 2008. *The Female Complaint.* Durham: Duke University Press.
Berlant, Lauren. 2011. *Cruel Optimism.* Durham: Duke University Press.
Berlant, Lauren, and Michael Warner. 1998. "Sex in Public." *Critical Inquiry* 24 (2): 547–566.
Berridge, Susan, and Karen Boyle. 2014. "I Love You, Man: Gendered Narratives of Friendship in Contemporary Hollywood Movies." *Feminist Media Studies* 14 (3): 353–368.
Brook, Barbara. 1999. *Feminist Perspectives on the Body.* 1st ed. London: Routledge.
Browne, Kath, and Catherine Nash. 2010. *Queer Methods and Methodologies: Intersecting Queer Theories and Social Science Research.* New York: Routledge.
Brundson, Charlotte. 1997. *Screen Tastes: Soap Opera to Satellite Dishes.* London: Routledge.
Burke, Phyliss. 1993. *Family Values: Two Moms and Their Son.* New York: Random House.
Butler, Judith. 1993. *Bodies That Matter: On the Discursive Limits of Sex.* London: Routledge.
Calhoun, Cheshire. 2000. *Feminism, Family, and the Politics of the Closet: Lesbian and Gay Displacement.* Oxford: Oxford University Press.
Campbell, Annily. 1999. *Childfree and Sterilized: Women's Decisions and Medical Responses.* London: Cassell.
Card, Claudia. 1995. *Lesbian Choices.* New ed. New York: Columbia University Press.
Carroll, Noel. 2005. *The Philosophy of Motion Pictures.* Hoboken, NJ: Wiley-Blackwell.

Cohen, Cathy J. 1997. "Punks, Bulldaggers, and Welfare Queens: The Radical Potential of Queer Politics?" *GLQ: A Journal of Lesbian and Gay Studies* 3 (4): 437–465.

Cook, Pam. 1998. "Duplicity in *Mildred Pierce*." In *Women and Film Noir*, edited by Anne Kaplan. London: British Film Institute.

Coontz, Stephanie. 2005. *Marriage, a History: How Love Conquered Marriage*. New York: Penguin Books.

Davitz, Lois. 1984. *Baby Hunger*. 1st ed. Minneapolis: Winston Press.

Doty, Alexander. 1993. *Making Things Perfectly Queer: Interpreting Mass Culture*. Minneapolis: University of Minnesota Press.

Doty, Alexander. 2002. *Flaming Classics: Queering the Film Canon*. New York: Routledge.

Doyle, Julia, and Karl Irmgard. 2008. "Shame on You: Cosmetic Surgery and Class Transformations in 10 Years Younger." In *Exposing Lifestyle Television: The Big Reveal*, edited by Gareth Palmer. Aldershot: Ashgate.

Duggan, Lisa. 2002. "The New Homonormativity: The Sexual Politics of Neoliberalism." In *Materializing Democracy*, edited by Russ Castronovo and Dana D. Nelson. Durham: Duke University Press.

Dyer, Richard. 1993. *The Matter of Images: Essays on Representations*. London: Routledge.

Dyer, Richard. 1997. *White*. London: Routledge.

Edelman, Lee. 2004. *No Future: Queer Theory and the Death Drive*. Durham: Duke University Press.

Edge, Brook Weihe. 2014. "Infertility on E! Assisted Reproductive Technologies and Reality Television." *Feminist Media Studies* 14 (5): 873–876.

Elsaesser, Thomas. 1973. "Film and the Novel: Reality and Realism of the Cinema." *Twentieth Century Studies* 9: 61.

Engels, Frederick. 2001. *The Origin of the Family, Private Property and the State*. London: Penguin.

Engwall, Kristina, and Helen Peterson. 2013. "Silent Bodies: Childfree Women's Gendered and Embodied Experiences." *European Journal of Women's Studies* 20 (4): 376–389.

Farquhar, Dion. 1996. *The Other Machine: Discourse and Reproductive Technologies*. London: Routledge.

Feasey, Rebecca. 2012. *From Happy Homemaker to Desperate Housewives: Motherhood and Popular Television*. London: Anthem Press.

Feasey, Rebecca. 2015. *Mothers on Mothers: Maternal Readings of Popular Television*. Edinburgh: Edinburgh University Press.

Feasey, Rebecca. 2017. "Good, Bad or Just Good Enough: Representations of Motherhood and the Maternal Role on the Small Screen." *Studies in the Maternal* 9 (1): 5, 1–31. https://doi.org/10.16995/sim.234.

Foucault, Michel. 1998. *The History of Sexuality: The Will to Knowledge: The Will to Knowledge*. Vol. 1. New ed. London: Penguin.

Franklin, Sarah. 1990. "Deconstructing 'Desperateness': The Social Construction of Infertility in Popular Representations of New Reproductive Technologies." In *The New Reproductive Technologies*, edited by Maureen McNeil. London: Palgrave Macmillan.

Friedman, May. 2014. "Unpacking MILF: Exploring Motherhood, Sexuality and Feminism." *Atlantis* 36 (2): 49–60.

Fuss, Diane. 2013. *Essentially Speaking: Feminism, Nature and Difference*. London: Routledge.

Gantz, Katherine. 2000. "'Not That There's Anything Wrong with That': Reading the Queer in Seinfeld." In *Straight With a Twist*, edited by Calvin Thomas. Champaign: University of Illinois Press.

Garland-Thomas, Rosmary. 2011. "Misfits: A Feminist Materialist Disability Concept." *Hypatia* 26 (3): 591–609. https://doi.org/10.1111/j.1527-2001.2011.01206.x.

Geraghty, Christine. 2003. "Aesthetics and Quality in Popular Television Drama." *International Journal of Cultural Studies* 6 (1): 25–45.

Gibbs, Anna. 2001. "Contagious Feelings: Pauline Hanson and the Epidemiology of Affect." *Australian Humanities Review* 24.

Gill, Rosalind. 2007. "Postfeminist Media Culture: Elements of Sensibility." *European Journal of Cultural Studies* 10 (2): 147–166.

Gillespie, Rosemary. 2003. "Childfree and Feminine Understanding the Gender Identity of Voluntarily Childless Women." *Gender & Society* 17 (1): 122–136.

Gillies, Val. 2006. *Marginalised Mothers: Exploring Working-Class Experiences of Parenting*. London and New York: Routledge.

Gledhill, Christine. 1987. "Speculations on the Relationship Between Soap Opera and Melodrama." *Quarterly Review of Film and Video* 14 (1–2): 103–124.

Gorton, Kristyn. 2008. "'There's No Place Like Home': Emotional Exposure, Excess and Empathy on TV." *Theatre, Film and Television* 1 (3): 3–15.

Gorton, Kristyn. 2009. *Media Audiences*. Edinburgh: Edinburgh University Press.

Griffin, Sean. 2009. *Hetero: Queering Representations of Straightness*. Albany: SUNY.

Griffin, Kate, and Lisa Mulholland. 1997. *Lesbian Motherhood in Europe*. London: Continuum Publishing.

Grossman, Julie. 2009. *Rethinking the Femme Fatale in Film Noir: Ready for Her Close-Up*. London: Palgrave Macmillan.

Halberstam, Judith. 2011. *The Queer Art of Failure*. Durham: Duke University Press.

Hanson, Helen. 2007. *Hollywood Heroines: Women in Film Noir and the Female Gothic Film*. New York: I.B. Taurus.

Hayes, Charlotte. 2013. *When Did White Trash Become the New Normal*. Washington, DC: Regnery Publishing.

Hewlett, Sylvia Anne. 2002. *Baby Hunger: The New Battle for Motherhood.* London: Atlantic.

Jeffreys, Sheila. 1986. *The Spinster and Her Enemies.* North Melbourne, VIC: Spinfex Press.

Klepfisz, Irena. 1999. "It Is Not a Child I Wish to Mother, It Is Myself." *Reproductive Health Matters* 7 (13): 96–102.

Kuhn, Annette. 1992. *Women's Pictures: Feminism and Cinema.* 2nd ed. London: Verso.

Lam, Carla. 2015. *New Reproductive Technologies and Disembodiment.* 1st ed. Abingdon: Routledge.

Lehr, Valerie.1999. *Queer Family Values: Debunking the Myth of the Nuclear Family.* Philadelphia: Temple University Press.

Lewin, Ellen. 1993. *Lesbian Mothers: Accounts of Gender in American Culture.* New York: Cornell University Press.

Littler, Jo, and Alison Winch. 2016. "Feminism and Childcare: A Roundtable with Sara de Benedictis, Gideon Burrows, Tracey Jensen, Jill Rutter and Victoria Showunmi." *Studies in the Maternal* 8 (1): 2. http://doi.org/10.16995/sim.212.

Loyo, Hilaria. 2007. "Blinding Blondes: Whiteness, Femininity, and Stardom." In *Questions of Colour in Cinema: From Paintbrush to Pixel*, edited by Wendy Everett. Oxford: Peter Lang.

McDonald, Jeffers. 2007. *Romantic Comedy: Boy Meets Girl Genre.* London: Wallflower.

Mckenna, Susan. 2002. "The Queer Insistence of Ally McBeal: Lesbian Chic, Postfeminism, and Lesbian Reception." *The Communication Review* 5 (4): 285–314.

McRobbie, Angela. 2004. "Post Feminism and Popular Culture." *Feminist Media Studies* 4 (3): 255–264.

Mills, Brett. 2009. *The Sitcom.* Edinburgh: Edinburgh University Press.

Moritz, Marguerite. 1987. "Coming Out Stories: The Creation of Lesbian Images on Prime Time TV." Paper presented at the Speech Communication Association Convention, Boston.

Moritz, Marguerite. 1999. "Old Strategies for New Texts: How American Television Is Creating and Treating Lesbian Characters." In *The Columbia Reader on Lesbian and Gay Men in Media, Society & Politics*, edited by Larry Gross and James D. Woods. New York: Columbia University Press.

Moseley, Rachel. 2003. *Growing Up with Audrey Hepburn: Text, Audience, Resonance.* Manchester: Manchester University Press.

Mumford, Laura. 1995. *Love and Ideology in the Afternoon: Soap Opera, Women, and Television Genre.* Bloomington: Indiana University Press.

Mustard, Deborah. 2000. "Spinster: An Evolving Stereotype Revealed Through Film." *Journal of Media Psychology*, 4: 1–9.

Neale, Stephen. 2000. *Genre and Hollywood*. London: Routledge.
O'Brien, Mary. 1983. *Politics of Reproduction*. New York: Routledge.
Oliver, Kelly. 2012. *Knock Me Up, Knock Me Down*. New York: Columbia University Press.
Park, Shelley. 2014. *Mothering Queerly, Queering Motherhood*. New York: State University of New York Press.
Peach, Lucinda Joy. 1998. *Women in Culture: A Women's Studies Anthology*. Oxford: Blackwell.
Peck, Janice. 1995. "TV Talk Shows as Therapeutic Discourse: The Ideological Labour of the Televised Talk Cure." *Communication Theory* 5 (1): 58–81.
Polikoff, Nancy. 1990. "This Child Does Have Two Mothers: Redefining Parenthood to Meet the Needs of Children in Lesbian Mother and Other Nontraditional Families." *The Georgetown Law Journal* 78: 459–575.
Probyn, Elspeth. 2005. *Blush: Faces of Shame*. Minneapolis: University of Minnesota Press.
Radway, Janice. 1983. "Women Read the Romance: The Interaction of Text and Context." *Feminist Studies* 9 (1): 53–78.
Radway, Janice. 1992. *Reading the Romance: Women, Patriarchy, and Popular Literature*. 2nd ed. Chapel Hill, NC: University North Carolina.
Rich, Adrienne. 1980. "Compulsory Heterosexuality and Lesbian Existence." *Signs: Journal of Women in Culture and Society* 5 (4): 631–660.
Roberts, Dorothy. 1996. "Race and the New Reproduction." *Faculty Scholarship at Penn Law.* 1154.
Rosenthal, Naomi. 2002. *Spinster Tales and Womanly Possibilities*. New York: SUNY Press.
Rules of Engagement. 2007–2013. "Audrey's Shower." Season 6, Episode 16. Directed by Ted Wass. Written by Tom Hertz and Vanessa McCarthy. TV programme. May 17, 2012. New York: CBS.
Sandelowski, Margarete. 1990. "Fault Lines: Infertility and Imperiled Sisterhood." *Feminist Studies* 16 (1): 33.
Sawicki, Janet. 1992. *Disciplining Foucault: Feminism, Power, and the Body*. New York: Routledge.
Sedgwick, Eve Kosofsky. 2003. *Touching Feeling: Affect, Pedagogy, Performativity*. New York: Duke University Press.
Sedgwick, Eve Kosofsky. 2008. *Epistemology of the Closet*. Berkeley: University of California Press.
Seidel, Linda. 2013. *Mediated Maternity and Popular Culture*. Lanham: Lexington.
Skeggs, Beverley. 1997. *Formations of Class and Gender: Becoming Respectable*. London: Sage.
Skeggs, Beverley, and Helen Wood. 2012. *Reacting to Reality Television, Performance, Audience and Value*. Oxon: Routledge.

Smith, Murray. 1995. *Engaging Characters: Fiction, Emotion and the Cinema*. Oxford: Clarendon Press.

Smith, Gregg. 1999. "Local Emotions, Global Moods and Film Structure." In *Passionate Views: Film, Cognition, and Emotion*, edited by Carl Plantinga and Greg Smith. Baltimore: John Hopkins University Press.

Sourbut, Elizabeth. 1996. "Gynogenesis: A Lesbian Appropriation of Reproductive Technologies." In *Between Monsters, Goddesses and Cyborgs: Feminist Confrontations with Science, Medicine and Cyberspace*, edited by Nina Lykke and Rosi Braidotti. London: Zed Books.

Sweeper, G. 1984. The Image of the Black Family and the White Family in American Primetime Television Programming 1970–1980. Doctoral dissertation. New York University, 1983. Dissertation Abstracts International. 44, 1964a.

Throsby, Karen. 2004. *When IVF Fails: Feminism, Infertility and the Negotiation of Normal*. Basingstoke: Palgrave.

Tincknell, Estella. 2005. *Mediating the Family: Gender, Culture and Representation*. London: Bloomsbury.

Tomkins, Silvan. 1992. *Affect, Imagery, Consciousness*. New York: Springer.

Tyler, Imogen. 2008. "Why the Maternal Now?" Published by the Department of Sociology, Lancaster University, Lancaster LA1 4YT, UK. http://www.lancs.ac.uk/fass/sociology/papers/tylerwhythematernalnow.pdf.

Walker, Janet. 1982. "Feminist Critical Practice: Female Discourse in Mildred Pierce." *Film Reader* 5: 164–172.

Walkerdine, Valerie. 1984. "Someday My Prince Will Come." In *Gender and Generation*, edited by Angela McRobbie and Misha Nava. London: Palgrave Macmillan.

Walkerdine, Valerie. 2011. "Shame on You! Intergenerational Trauma and Working Class Femininity on Reality Television." In *Reality Television and Class*, edited by Helen Wood and Beverly Skeggs. London: BFI.

Walks, Michelle. 2007. "Breaking the Silence: Infertility, Motherhood, and Queer Culture." *Journal of the Motherhood Initiative for Research and Community Involvement* 9 (2): 130–143.

Weber, Brenda. 2009. *Makeover TV: Selfhood, Citizenship, and Celebrity*. Durham: Duke University Press.

Weston, Kath. 1991. *Families We Choose*. 1st ed. New York: Columbia University Press.

Willemen, Paul. 1971. "Distanciation and Douglas Sirk." *Screen* 12 (2): 63–67.

Williams, Linda. 1991. "Film Bodies: Gender, Genre, and Excess." *Film Quarterly* 44 (4): 2–13.

Winch, Alison. 2012. "We Can Have It All." *Feminist Media Studies* 12 (1): 69–82.

Wittig, Monique. 1992. *The Straight Mind: And Other Essays*. Boston: Beacon Press.

CHAPTER 5

Queer Futures: Chosen Families and Alternative Intimacies

The texts that have been discussed throughout the analytical chapters, and which will be revisited in this chapter, are *Coronation Street*, *Giuliana & Bill*, *Rules of Engagement*, *The New Normal* and *Baby Mama*. Other popular cultural texts will also be referred to, to illuminate key points.

The primary focus of this chapter is to acknowledge and explore the focus groups' resistance to the dominant narratives of motherhood and family in the texts, through their varying positions in relation to motherhood. Furthermore, their reflexivity to genre techniques will also be discussed, particularly through their desire for more alternative happy endings that don't depend on the arrival of a genetic child. The participants' acknowledgment of different forms of love, outside of the genetic tie and mother–child bond will also be discussed. Throughout this chapter I argue that the cultural articulations of love and family in relation to the surrogacy storylines are problematic for the participants in my study, and thus result in resistant readings of the texts.

This chapter is divided into three parts. "Normal Service Has Resumed" explores the participants' desire for alternative happy endings and more tolerant cultural articulations of identities outside of natural notions of motherhood, where babies are conceived through heterosexual sex, without the use of reproductive technologies. "It Must Be Love" unpicks the myth of blood ties and the mother–child bond through a

L. Le Vay, *Surrogacy and the Reproduction of Normative Family on TV*, Palgrave Studies in Science and Popular Culture,
https://doi.org/10.1007/978-3-030-17570-2_5

discussion of the wider range of love connections outside of the traditional family unit, and "Queering Kinship" explores the possibilities of new family structures built on these connections to provide transcending counter-narratives of family, for future cultural articulations. A range of queer theory, emotion and affect and race and reproduction scholarship will be drawn on to underpin the analysis.

Normal Service Has Resumed

> I think it's interesting why they [the infertile protagonists] have to get pregnant too at the end. It's as if people can't quite cope with the idea of women who can't have children.
>
> (Carrie, mixed mothers focus group, 2015)

As explored in Chapter 4, the female characters struggling with infertility in *Baby Mama* and *Rules of Engagement* are portrayed as incomplete as women, until they become positioned as normative by becoming natural mothers and situated within a heterosexual couple dyad. Carrie's statement above suggests that most audiences, or 'people', would struggle with an ending that isn't conventionally happy, where the disruption in the narrative (infertility) hasn't been restored, fixed, through heterosexual romance and the formation of the normative biological family unit. Carrie's response also implies that she, as a viewer, is situated against the mainstream, which infers a resistance to the texts.

A discussion between Carrie, Sonja, Carla and Jackie (mixed mothers focus group) further indicates a displeasure of viewing these happy endings in the texts:

> Sonja: They're saying it's better if you do it yourself.
> Carla: Yeah, I think it's reinforcing that it's natural and normal to have children.
> Sonja: In a natural and normal way.
> Carla: It shows you how the story went, but the final point is to reinforce… see that, enjoy that, but this is the message.
> Sonja: Yes, but don't worry, normal service has been resumed.
> Jackie: Yeah, it ends up being conventional.
> Sonja It's a bit of a cop out really, isn't it?
>
> (Carrie, Sonja, Carla and Jackie, mixed mothers focus group, 2015)

In addition to demonstrating an annoyance with how both *Baby Mama* and *Rules of Engagement* conclude, this discussion also illuminates how female audiences are active, and not passive, in being able to reject a dominant narrative within a text (Ang 1985; Fiske 1989; Radway 1983; Skeggs and Wood 2008; Stacey 1993). However, in doing so, it is clear that the participants are also displaying a recognition and understanding of how the function of the happy ending is an integral part of the genre's narrative, to provide pleasure to the audience through fantasy. Or, as Kelly Oliver (2012) argues, to quell anxieties 'with reassuring tales of white career women getting babies before it's too late' (2012, 18). As Carrie stated: 'people can't quite cope with the idea of women who can't have children'.

In addition, Rachel (non-mother's focus group) was also able to identify the genre mechanisms of the sitcom and the mom-com, in relation to the viewing experience and the happy ending: 'People watch those shows for a reason, they want that ending before they've even sat down to the opening credits'. Ien Ang (1995) argues that the happy ending is integral to the feminisation of genre, which provides pleasure through an escape into fantasy, which both Lauren Berlant (2008) and Janice Radway (1983, 1992) also claim aims to transport the female viewer into an imagined world, a distraction from the reality of everyday life. Furthermore, Rachel's statement resonates with Kirstyn Gorton's (2009) argument that some female viewers select texts of a certain genre based on how they *want* to respond emotionally, such as 'preparing for a good cry' (2009, 129). However, as evidenced in the above discussion, not all viewers find pleasure, or escape—the participants are irritated, arguing that such endings are 'a cop out' and 'conventional'. I propose that inferring that 'normal service' is resumed through the narrative closure of natural pregnancy suggests that comfort can be found in what is being presented as the utopia of normativity (Berlant 2008). As the participants' responses indicate, such a presumption of what is deemed normative and happy does not take into consideration a range of possible narrative outcomes that might be received positively by audiences. As Laura (non-mothers focus group) expressed through her displeasure in how the childless characters were portrayed, in relation to the happy ending:

> It's great that these fictional characters can get pregnant, but it's kind of a shame that it can't be left as you can't have kids, you know what I mean? That happens. There really are people who can't have kids and they don't

> get pregnant even if they try, and it doesn't just happen. Be good if they just left it… it would be interesting if someone wrote that into a story instead of doing the nice Hollywood ending.
>
> (Laura, non-mothers focus group, 2015)

What is interesting about Laura's statement is that she describes the happy endings in the texts as 'Hollywood' endings, which shows how she is reading the endings in relation to the cliché and convention of a specific genre, one that has been, as claimed by James MacDowell (2013), constant, persistent and ubiquitous in conventional cinema. As he proposes: 'It is not simply that most Hollywood films have interchangeable "happy endings," but that *all* do' (2013, 3). It can be suggested that these happy endings are shaped through what Judith Butler calls a 'heterosexual imperative' (1993, 2) which is where norms work to enforce sexual difference as a method of regulation. In this case, the norms of heterosexual family. Pamela Demory and Christopher Pullen (2013) claim that in the context of the heterosexual imperative in classic Hollywood cinema romance drives the story *and* offers a closure that 'restores the couple or family unit (in the "happy ending") or fails to restore "normal" order (in the unhappy or open ending)' (2013, 1).

It has been widely argued, particularly through feminist and queer theory—as touched upon in the previous chapter—that the happy ending, which is rooted in myths and fairy tales, is perpetuated in popular culture through a compulsory heterosexuality that packages happiness within the heteronormative (Ahmed 2010; Franklin 1990; Halberstam 2011; Rich 1980). As Kathleen Barry (1985) argues, heterosexual romance embedded in the storylines of TV and film is a Western concept and universal ideology that sets out to indoctrinate women from an early age. However, as is evident in the audience data, it doesn't work on *all* women.[1]

Sara Ahmed (2010) has identified the heteronormative shaping of narratives as what is constructed as a heterosexual happiness, which suggests that 'heterosexual love becomes about the possibility of a happy ending; about what life is aimed toward, as well as being what gives life direction, a purpose, or as what drives the story' (2010, 90). The happy endings in the texts indicate compliance to hetero-norms, which through the flow of the narrative structure reposition the infertile characters as normative. This is facilitated through the final equilibrium of natural pregnancy and heterosexual love. By staying on the heteronormative path, it has been proposed that these characters, like the homosexual characters in *The New Normal*, are rewarded with happiness for remaining in the approximation to, or moving towards, signs of straightness—pregnancy, family, heterosexual romance (Ahmed 2006, 2010). As Ahmed (2010) identifies in her analysis of TV movie, *If These Walls Could Talk 2*, where sperm donation has enabled the happy ending of pregnancy for a lesbian couple, 'the promise of the child becomes the promise of happiness' (2010, 113–114). It is the promise of happiness wrapped up in the arrival of the *future foetus* that drives the narratives in all of the texts in focus, regardless of the gendered pairing of the parents. As the representations suggest, as long as there are two (white) parents, settled within a monogamous, loving relationship and preferably married—'straight! gay! Over 65! doesn't matter!' (Briggs 2017, 125)—then the reward of happiness is reaped through the production of a genetic child.

In all of the texts that have been explored that feature female characters struggling with infertility—Izzy in *Coronation Street*, Giuliana in *Giuliana & Bill*, Audrey in *Rules of Engagement* and Kate in *Baby Mama*—the ultimate goal, and final equilibrium, regardless of genre, is the acquisition of the genetic child, preferably through normative heterosexual sex within the romance narrative. As pinpointed by Rhian (pre-mothers focus group) in her discussion of *Baby Mama*, but which applies to all of these characters in the texts regardless of whether they had a partner or not, they 'wanted a child to love'. This desire eclipses the romantic love narrative in favour of maternal fulfilment.[2] In addition, this narrative also shapes popular constructions of infertility (Franklin 1990). Heterosexual romance is necessary, but it's not the narrative's primary drive. As further illuminated by Laura (non-mothers focus group), the narrative closure of these stories is natural conception, which she felt was not representative, or tolerant, of the complexities of fertility that affect women (and men) in the real world. As she stated: 'There really are people who can't have kids and they don't get pregnant even if they try'. This attachment to reproducing the genetic child demonstrates the fetishist fixation of heteronormativity which places heterosexual procreative relations above all other forms of sexual expression (Barrett and McIntosh 1991; Edelman 2003).

Although Lee Edelman (2003) claims, persuasively, that in the context of right-wing social and political beliefs, queers, feminists and pro-abortionists are to blame for future reproductive ruin, he has made an error by omitting the threat of female heterosexual infertility as he automatically ascribes women to the 'site of the unqueer' (Halberstam 2011, 119). This association of women with biological reproduction is essentialist. In addition, Edelman also disregards same-sex familial desires as assimilationist, rather than having the potential for resistance (Ahmed 2006; Calhoun 2000). The notion of challenging norms through gay marriage and family will be explored towards the end of this chapter. Drawing on the audience data and the textual analysis I argue that the infertile woman is being portrayed as a 'reproductive misfit' (Lam 2015, 112)—a threat to the heterosexual reproductive future through the non-production of genetic children. In the cultural articulations under analysis, reproductive technologies—such as surrogate pregnancies enabled by embryo transfer—have become a tool by which to enable loving couples only, straight and gay, acculturation into the acceptable heterosexual mainstream.

At this juncture, it is important to re-emphasise that the appropriation of the signifier *queer* and queer politics by heterosexuals to critique the heteronormative can be seen as problematic. Suzanna Walters (1996) argues, justifiably, that a heterosexual queer position is one of privilege, which she finds disturbing as it is not defined by sexual choice or gay identity, but a desire to identify with a broader concept of queer that denotes the non-normative. As I have previously stated, drawing on Kath Browne and Catherine J. Nash (2010), adopting a queer lens for research is useful as it can expose deeply entrenched meanings and related power structures, which I believe I have done so throughout this thesis. Furthermore, it is important to reiterate that queer is a verb that has been mobilised in these discussions to not *identify* as queer, but to explore similarities between queer subjectivity and heterosexual infertility, while also challenging what is being constructed in these texts as normative. As argued by Annette Schlichter (2004) drawing on Butler, the term can 'express an affiliation with anti-homophobic politics' *and* critique and subvert 'the practices of heteronormative normalization' (2004, 547) which in this project describes heterosexuals who are not complying to normative practices of family and reproduction.

This notion of non-compliance can be identified through how Sally (mixed mothers focus group) was able to recognise how normative family and female fulfilment through motherhood is constructed in the texts' narratives is also reproduced in her own lived experience as a single, white, middle-class, heterosexual, childless woman in her early forties:

> A while back I was at a drinks party with some older people, and they were like: "So, are you married?" No. "Got a partner?" No. "Any children?" No. I was like: "hello! You know, actually my name is Sally, and would you like to learn something about *me* rather than these add-ons?"
>
> (Sally, mixed mothers focus group, 2015)

Sally's experience demonstrates how her identity is viewed by social peers as incomplete, which is also reflected in the work of Irena Klepfisz (1999). Klepfisz argues that dominant notions of what it means to be a 'woman' are myths, created through cultural mediation, that are hard to escape from in daily interactions with individuals and structures:

> This is a powerful myth that is nurtured by everything around us, fostered by the media, by popular literature, by parents, by questionnaires we fill out for jobs... Are you married? No. Do you live alone? Yes. How many members in your household? One. It is a myth perpetually reinforced by the assumption that only family and children provide us with a purpose and place. Bestow upon us an honour, respect, love, and comfort. (1999, 97)

This resonates with the earlier argument that the heterosexual romance narrative is prolific throughout popular culture, and that motherhood and normative family is constructed in everyday life to provide refuge through convention. As Carla (mixed mothers focus group) claimed in the previous chapter, the happy endings in these texts isolated her, rather than as has been suggested, made her feel a sense of belonging (Berlant 2008). For her, there was no point of identification, as they created 'this kind of stick we are supposed to be beating ourselves with'.

Reproductive technologies, therefore, through this core narrative, do not symbolise liberation from reproduction, which Shulamith Firestone (1970) claimed would make women more fulfilled and equal to men, but quite the opposite. The driving narrative in these texts suggest that to find fulfilment as a woman is *within* and not *outside* of the normative folds of natural motherhood and the conventional family structure. The articulations of reproductive technologies in these representations do not exhibit the potential to dismantle the biological, nuclear family, as many feminists argued Firestone hoped for, but aims to build and reinforce it, ignited through the fear of *no future*. However, it has been suggested, through Deborah Halbert's (2004) attentive reading of *The Dialectic of Sex* (1970), that Firestone did in fact infer that reproductive technologies *also* had the potential to subordinate women, rather than liberate.

Halbert proposes that Firestone indicated it was the underlying gender roles within the family structure and normative expectations of the woman as mother and child-bearer that needed to be challenged. As she argues, Firestone was implying that: 'Technology alone will not liberate women and men, instead there must be a transformation in the way sex-roles are understood, a transformation that can only take place if technology is used to give women choices other than childrearing' (in Merck and Sandford 2010, 31). This argument resonates with Dorothy Robert's (1996) claim that 'rather than disrupt the stereotypical family, they [reproductive technologies] enable couples to create one' (1996, 936).

Films and TV shows radiate dreams and fantasies, and in some texts, for some audiences, authentic representations. However, as highlighted by the focus group participants, they also show inauthentic portrayals, which arouse discomfort, rather than comfort. The audience data suggests that although it was perceived as positive to see characters that *do* become pregnant naturally, there should be representational space to accommodate alternative happy endings that don't have to rely on such conventional narrative conclusions. The participants wanted to see more realistic and positive storylines and portrayals of women outside expectations and experiences of motherhood, which are complex. This includes exposing the myth of the mother/child bond, which the mothers in the focus groups claim isn't always love at first sight, as is depicted in the texts.

It Must Be Love

> I find it a real falsehood… it didn't happen to me, and I know everybody's different, but there's this mythology, that these shows perpetuate, that when you see your baby, you fall in love.
>
> (Carrie, mixed mothers focus group, 2015)

Across the majority of narratives that feature the birth of a child, regardless of genre, there is a love-at-first-sight moment between the mother and baby, even if the pregnancy was unwanted, or uncomfortable, and regardless of whether the child is born with or without a genetic connection. Drawing on Oliver's (2012) work on pregnancy in Hollywood film, this 'love spell' is due to the growing romanticism of conception and pregnancy within the mom-com genre. These moments in the narrative suggest that a woman finally becomes whole, completed. As Rachel (non-mothers focus group) declared in response to what she believed the texts were saying: 'You're not a real woman until you've had a child'.

However, the compulsory love spell between the mother and genetic child, as has been recognised by mothers in the focus groups, is not always reflective of real life. As Carrie (mixed mothers focus group) explained in relation to her own experience as a mother: 'it didn't happen to me'. Carrie and Sonja (mixed mothers focus group) also had a revealing discussion about the mother–child bond, which further dismantles the fantasy of the maternal love spell that drives the narratives:

> Carrie: That wasn't my experience.
> Sonja: It wasn't mine, either.
> Carrie: I was just so tired… I know I'm not supposed to say that.
> Sonja: It's definitely a gradual process. Well, it was for me.
> Carrie: It's mythologising this bond with the baby, which it might be for some women, but I think for a lot of women it isn't.
> Sonja: I'm really glad you said that, as before I had my son, I read a book… luckily, I read lots of books… and at least one of them said that if you don't get overwhelmed with maternal love when you first see your child, then don't worry, it comes in in different ways, and at different paces for people, so don't panic. I was convinced I wouldn't be one of those weirdos that… and I wasn't. But, it was definitely a process that started about two days in, and then grew and grew and grew… and then in the end you're besotted.
> Lulu: So, do you think that the romance in these shows is between the mother and the baby?
> Carrie: Yeah. We don't see the surrogate or the mother going "take it away for God's sake!" do we?
>
> (Carrie, Sonja and Lulu, mixed mothers focus group, 2015)

This above discussion infers that the notion of falling in love with your baby at first sight is a myth, perpetuated by such representations. We see this happening in *Waitress* (2007), where diner employee Jenna discovers she is pregnant when she leaves an abusive marriage. She is so distraught about the pregnancy she names a pie after it, the 'Bad Baby Pie'. When the baby girl arrives, Jenna falls in love with her immediately. She no longer has the husband, but she has the baby. In mom-com *What to Expect When You're Expecting* (2012), character Wendy is in discomfort throughout her entire pregnancy. She constantly chases the facial baby glow of pregnancy, the one that as she declares, 'they promise you on the cover of those magazines'. At the film's conclusion, she finds it not radiating from her complexion, but wrapped in the baby in her arms.[3] I propose that these narratives are perpetuating a pro-life agenda through what the research findings have indicated is a culturally constructed myth of the baby–mother bond, the baby representing a future full of hope, promise, happiness, and the good life to come (Ahmed 2010; Berlant 1994; Edelman 2003).

The texts that have been discussed throughout this thesis include similar scenes. Tina, the surrogate in *Coronation Street*, bonds with baby Jake moments after giving birth, despite not being genetically related to him, 'I fell in love with him, when I held him… I thought he was mine, part of me'. The love spell of the mother–baby union also appears in *Rules of Engagement*, *Baby Mama*, *Giuliana & Bill* and *The New Normal*, with the two dads *and* the surrogate being portrayed as being weak-at-the-knees. The only character shown to have no maternal feelings towards the baby is Brenda, the lesbian surrogate in *Rules of Engagement*.

What is evident in this discussion is that both Carrie and Sonja shared feelings of shame for admitting their experiences did not mirror those represented in the texts. These feelings are identified through comments such as 'I know I'm not supposed to say that', 'I'm really glad you said that…' and 'I was convinced I wouldn't be one of those weirdos…' These responses reflect a similar stance to that of Carla, a childless participant in the same group who also struggled to relate to the texts' narratives and character constructions. Furthermore, Carrie and Sonja's responses also reflect the feelings of isolation, deviancy and shame that have been identified in the representations of the childless characters, particularly Audrey in *Rules of Engagement*, as discussed in Chapter 4. Sonja's response to these texts reveals a similar position. The 'weirdo' as she described in this context is not the infertile woman, but the woman who does not form an immediate bond with her child. These findings resonate with those of Tina Miller (2005) whose interviews with new mothers revealed feelings of guilt and shame. The women in her study modified their birth narratives, from bad to good, in fear of being judged if they were to admit the experience didn't go to plan, and that the bonding with the newborn wasn't immediate.

Carrie and Sonja are both mothers in monogamous relationships. Like the childless characters that are shamed through genre devices, both Carrie and Sonja, as viewers, have also been shamed, excluded from the narrative by what is being culturally presented as expected social norms. It is interesting to highlight here the possibility that the 'weirdo' could be describing Brenda in *Rules of Engagement*, despite Carrie's assertion that none of the intended mothers or surrogates were shown as rejecting the babies at birth. During the birth scene, Brenda was shown as being more interested in the ordeal being over and cracking open a beer than gazing lovingly at the baby. 'Weirdo' applied in this context, therefore, can be read as reinforcing the notion that lesbianism and motherhood are socially and culturally incompatible.

The love bond between the mother and baby that is constructed in the texts is shaped through a fairy tale narrative, much like the narrative of romantic love that dominates the texts. It can be argued that this ideal of love endorses a set of norms that do not reflect social reality, particularly in relation to heterosexual communities, as the traditional family unit is breaking down. This is evident in soaring divorce rates, spouse abuse, abandonment and promiscuity (Evans 2003; Weston 1991). Families are being combined, and extended familial relationships formed.

Drawing on studies of gay and lesbian family formations and poor black urban communities, these new formations can be described as fictive, or chosen families. These extended kinship networks reach beyond the boundaries of the nuclear family unit, to be explored in more detail below. What these formations of family evidence, which is not made visible in the representations under discussion, is that love, as a concept, is more complex and elastic than is being articulated. Love can describe the feelings that drive heterosexual sexual partnerships with the primary aim to procreate, viewed as 'kinship's ultimate referent' (Weston 1991, 33). Love can also describe close bonds with persons with no genetic tie, as well as deep connections to animals and even the joy of material objects, and the experience of sensory pleasures such as taste, touch, smell and sound. As Mary Evans (2003) explains:

> We love ice cream just as much as we might love our cat or the person we live with. We are, as people in our culture – very active as 'lovers' of objects, situations and even people. But the extent to which the same word is used to cover a multitude of possibilities should also warn us of the conceptual confusion around the idea. It is possible, therefore, that we love too much and too widely and that we have reached a situation where it is difficult to distinguish between different types of love, and the different contexts in which we might love. (2003, 22)

It is possible to suggest, then, that this notion of loving too much, and this cultural obsession with love and the genetic tie, can make way for a range of other positive emotions which fictive kinship can be built on—such as support, intimacy and friendship (Rubin 1993; Weston 1991). Meaningful family structures can be *made* that undermine the nuclear biological unit, not to be viewed socially, culturally or politically as false, or lesser than this elevated ideal (Calhoun 2000; Carsten 2004).

It has been proposed that the cultural constructions of love in mainstream texts, such as those under discussion, have been composed to offer female audiences a sense of belonging in the social world through the sentimentality of romantic love—the loss of which being unimaginable (Berlant 2008; Evans 2003). As Evans (2003) queries: 'Is love an emotion or an expectation? Dare we entertain a world without love and could another vocabulary, in which words such as care, commitment and desire were more often used, actually make us happier?' (2003, 2–3). A line delivered by *Coronation Street* character, ladies' underwear machinist Beth Tinker, who is horrified at the surrogate arrangement, provoked discussion within the focus groups. During a scene in the local pub the Rovers Return, where the surrogate Tina eventually returned to work, Beth whispers to her drinking partner across the table: 'You never know what love is until you've had a kid'. Paula, Rebecca, Laura and Rachel (non-mothers focus group) had a lively debate:

> Paula: You *can* love someone who's not your child.
> Rebecca: You can love a pet; you can love another human being.
> Laura: I think it's a different type of love.
> Rachel: Yeah, I agree with that.
> Rebecca: Yeah, a different type of love, *but* I think that comment sounds a bit superficial.
> Laura: It's verging into the superiority complex of mothers, that patronising kind of "you won't understand".
> Rachel: But… who's that directed at? Because there are fathers in the world… Do you hear fathers saying that they've never loved anyone like that, when they've left their kids and not paid any maintenance? I don't think they'd agree with that. So, again, it's an idea of what a woman should be thinking.
> (Paula, Rebecca, Laura and Rachel, non-mothers focus group, 2015)

This discussion reflects on, and in doing so rejects, the myth of the mother and child bond, which infers that childless women are incapable of experiencing maturity, to be responsible or have the ability to truly care, if they haven't had a child. This upholds and perpetuates dominant notions of femininity that suggest that to be a mother is to be natural, womanly, whole. The non-mothers in this group believe that the love they can feel for other human beings, or for pets, can be just as meaningful, while recognising that this form of love is a 'different type of love'. What has also been identified is the gendering of the concept of love as being central to women's experience, which is constructed in popular texts and performed through female identities (Berlant 2008; Evans 2003). As Rachel highlights through identifying the gendered differences between the mother and father roles, in relation to the love bond with a child: 'it's an idea of what a woman should be thinking'.

Other participants, including the mothers, also rejected this statement. Not only did the mothers share the reality that women don't always love their own children (Carrie: 'It's that whole mythology around maternal love… you can hate them more than any other person'), but both mothers and non-mothers talked about the love they felt, and still feel, for pets, stepfamily and friends' children, and that the feelings associated with love are not, as has been constructed in the texts, so inflexible, fixed, but which have many shades. Sonja was able to describe how love as a feeling mutated in relation to how she felt about her partner, her horses and her son. Although she recognised the love for her child as being powerful, Sonja also empathised with and related to Jackie, who has no children, and is bisexual. Jackie shared the feelings of love she felt for her nieces, and her friends' children:

> Jackie: Well, I feel that about my nieces, and kids that I've looked after for eight years.
> Sonja: I actually felt like that about horses I looked after when I was a kid.
> Jackie: I love them to death.
> Sonja: And that you'll always love them, and nothing would ever stop you from loving them.
> Jackie: Even when technically they aren't my kids.
> (Sonja and Jackie, mixed mothers focus group, 2015)

This illustrates that bonds of love can, and are, formed with a range of beings, animal and human, with no biological or romantic connection.

The relationship between animals and humans, as illustrated by Sonja's love of her horses when she was a child, is particularly revealing. This love attachment to animals, which has been noted as acutely strong in relation to horses (Birke and Hockenhull 2012, 2016; Charles 2014, 2016; Charles and Davies 2008; Smart 2011), shows how animals become deeply embedded within family lives. Nickie Charles (2014) has described these human–animal kinship bonds a 'multi-species household' (2014, 12). Charles has proposed such kinship structures can be called a post-human family, where humans and animals co-habit—animals considered valued family members (Charles 2014; Fudge 2008; Haraway 2007). This exchange between Jackie and Sonja also demonstrates how women from different subject positions, situated on opposing sides of the binary—heterosexual/lesbian, mother/non-mother—are able to relate to each other's experiences of meaningful love bonds, which indicates the potential for a coalition politics which will be explored in Chapter 6.

The findings in the audience data infer, in opposition to what is being portrayed in the texts under analysis, that deep love connections can be developed with a range of subjects, across a range of communities, that do not have to rely so obsessively on the genetic tie. As Michael Warner (1999) and Judith Halberstam (2011) suggest, straight culture can learn from gay culture; in this context, particularly through the intervention of reproductive technologies that can bend and reshape the contours of family. Interestingly, this reveals a tension—reproductive technologies can be used to reinforce normative heterosexual families as well as make them. As Warner argues: 'against assimilation, one could insist that the dominant culture assimilate to queer culture, not the other way around. Straight culture has already learned much from queers, and it shouldn't stop now' (1999, 74).

Queering Kinship

> I'm very open-minded about the family and all its permutations, but I still think that our society isn't very tolerant. It may become more normalised over time, but right now I think it's quite difficult.
>
> (Carrie, mixed mothers focus group, 2015)

Although Carrie was responding to how the narratives in the texts concluded through the normalisation of the family unit, her comment was also referring to how same-sex parenting must be construed to become accessible, due to social and cultural intolerances to identities and practices of family outside of the heteronormative, as discussed in Chapter 3. What is important to highlight here, is how such intolerances have been integral to the resignifications of family (Butler 1993) that have emerged through gay and black communities, which, I argue, drawing on Warner (1999), straight culture could learn from.

Historically, gay and black communities have created an alternative version of family to create bonds between social and political allies, but which have also strengthened communities, for survival. For example, gay communities in the 1980s developed new family connections through the impact of AIDS, by caring for the dying (Calhoun 2000; Weston 1991), and also through new articulations of kinship which surfaced through ball culture in America, an underground drag scene that emerged in Harlem as far back as 1869, but which became more visible in the 1930s (Chauncey 1995). Initially a space for white gay men to socialise, ball culture later became popular within black and Latino LGTBQ communities in the 1960s–1970s by providing a safe environment, and a space of resistance, at a time when homophobic hate crime was rife. With a strong link to high fashion and dance music, ball culture became more visible, globally, through artists such as Madonna, whose hit record *Vogue* (1990) brought the scene's dance style 'voguing' to mainstream culture. The same year the now critically acclaimed documentary *Paris Is Burning* (1990) was released, which captured ball culture in 1980s New York. The film encapsulated how the LGTBQ community of primarily blacks and Latinos expressed their identities in response to the white, heterosexual and middle-class mainstream.

Within ball culture 'houses' were created to symbolise family structures. These new families acted as a support network for the LGBTQ community, many of whom were African American youth affected by HIV/AIDS,[4] who had been ejected from their homes (Arnold and Bailey 2009). These 'house' categories were headed by the figure of the drag 'mother', who would mentor the newcomers, the 'children', and often provide them with a home and shelter. In her analysis of *Paris Is Burning* and ball culture, Judith Butler (1993) argues that the resignification of kinship relations is 'not a vain or useless imitation, but the social and discursive building of community, a community that binds, cares and teaches, that shelters and enables' (1993, 137). Ball culture, she claims, is the frame that houses these new sets of kinship relations.

Ball culture is not central to this discussion, so cannot be explored in depth. However, its structure as a community is important to mobilise in relation to the emergence of alternative formations of family, through the resignification of family categories, and how these responses to normative discourses are problematic. Butler (1993) claims that through the appropriation and redeployment of these terms, kinship relations can be reformed that function as an oppositional discourse, which exhibits the potential to transcend the traditional family unit through a subversion of norms. However, it can be suggested that even through a reinterpretation of family, the dominant hierarchical, heteronormative structure is still imposed. This is a pattern that has also been identified in the formation of same-sex parenting and marriage, where family structures have been modelled on heterosexual norms such as lifelong monogamy, rituals and heterosexual romance (Folger 2008), as discussed in Chapter 3. I argue, drawing on the audience data, that a wider range of alternative family structures must be recognised, that illustrate a critical rethinking of family that involves a network of friends and family in a 'plurality of intimate and familial norms' (Calhoun 2000).

Through the long history of black communities in America, extended kinship structures have been formed to act as familial networks, not just for emotional support, but for the pooling of resources to survive. What materialised through these communities was a counter-narrative of family, also recognised in the drag families of ball culture. Terms such as 'sister' and 'brother' were appropriated by feminism during the Civil Rights Movement as a mark of respect for political allies; terms that were initially employed within black communities as a gesture of racial solidarity to make meaningful—make as *real* as blood ties—non-biological connections. As Roberts (1996) claims: 'blood ties are less significant to the definition of family in the Black community than they have traditionally been for white America' (1996, 214).

The complexities of this appropriation into white feminist culture are important, specifically in relation to the notion of extended kinships networks. It is important to emphasise that these terms are implicit to black culture. As civil rights activist Pat Rosezelle (1995) outlines, the origin of the sister/brother terms are a legacy from slavery, when as the result of the fragmentation of families, new families were built; new allegiances and bonds formed. As she argues: 'When people are bastardized, raped, and fragmented from their families, they have to create a family' (in Friedman and Weiss 1995, 139). Furthermore, Rosezelle emphasises that 'sister' and 'brother' are not only terms of respect—which signify community, solidarity and affection—but are used as a political act, to acknowledge a connection to those who have been disrespected through racism.

It is understandable that the appropriation of these revised kinship terms by white culture, particularly white feminism, can be viewed as problematic despite good intentions, through the imbalance of power and privilege (Lugones and Rosezelle 1995).[5] However, while acknowledging this, the notion of 'fictive kin' is useful to mobilise in the discussion of alternative family formations, which includes non-biological family memberships within gay communities. Kath Weston (1991) describes these alternative family memberships as 'chosen families' (1991, 116) which she argues is a concept that aims to act as a contrast to heterosexual biological units.

However, as Calhoun (2000) correctly points out, such formations are derived from the fictive kinship of historical black culture, and which also 'characterizes the reality of many heterosexual families who fail in various ways to construct a nuclear family around a procreative married couple' (2000, 150). However, through the utilisation of these structures it is imperative to emphasise there is no intention to retract from the tenor of their origins, but they have been employed to illustrate how family structures can, and have, functioned in meaningful ways, in different forms, outside of the convention of genetic ties, which are rendered invisible in these texts.

Extended kinship structures and meaning attached to non-genetic bonds of love have emerged as significant to all of the focus group participants, regardless of their differing positions to motherhood. Even the younger group of women recognised the value of kinship outside of the genetic bond. As Rhian (pre-mothers focus group) stated: 'I don't think it matters if you give birth to the child or not, even when you adopt a child you love it as much as if you've given birth to it. I think it's about your mindset, and how you love them as they grow up'.

Tara (non-mothers focus group) talked about how meaningful bonds were formed through the breaking up of her once normative family unit, into a new, alternative shaped family structure:

> I love my stepbrother even though he's not... and I say he's my brother. And he doesn't look like me, but I always say: "yeah, he's my brother". It's how you form bonds and love people.
>
> (Tara, non-mothers focus group, 2015)

Tara described the love she feels for her stepbrother, with the same value as if he were a blood-related brother, regardless of there being no family resemblance. She regards her love for him as real. Tara's example demonstrates the reality of heterosexual families that re-form through combining families post-divorce or separation, which results in an extended family that features a mixture of genetic and non-genetic relations (Calhoun 2000; Park 2014; Weston 1991). This also applies to the re-structuring of the nuclear family when a parent comes out as gay.

These revised family structures disassemble long-established notions articulated through popular culture, politics and law that infer that biological ties are associated with straight families (real families, normative), which positions non-genetic family formations as weaker (unreal, non-normative), such as chosen families within the black and gay communities (Park 2014). However, interestingly, with the growing popularity of same-sex couples opting for surrogacy arrangements, having a genetic connection is still not enough to assimilate into the normative, as has been shown through the discussion of the texts—natural pregnancy through heterosexual love having been identified as the most desired outcome. As the recent changes in surrogacy laws in India and Thailand have dictated, only heterosexual couples now need apply. Gay couples and single persons are prohibited from the process. It is important to highlight that it is only a short time ago that same-sex relationships have been recognised by the legal system. Homosexuals and lesbians are still excluded from marriage in some countries, and as Cheshire Calhoun (2000) has emphasised, not long ago gay and lesbian parents have been viewed by the courts as harmful to children.[6]

The invisibility of extended and/or chosen families in these texts' narratives exposes a core anxiety of a woman remaining uncoupled and childless. The concern surrounding this outcome expresses the fear that reproductive technologies are separating sex from reproduction *and* that the biological nuclear family unit is under threat, due to the more alternative kinship structures that are becoming continually more visible socially yet are not being articulated through mainstream contemporary culture. This is evident in the construction of familial norms in relation to the genetic connection, the purification and preservation of whiteness and white privilege, and the heterosexual romance narrative, which shapes all of the texts in focus.

Where Oliver (2012) has proposed that the anxieties of separating sex from reproduction are placated by narratives bringing them back together,

I argue, inspired by the audience data, that we have now witnessed a further shift, that narratives are attempting to reconcile the breakdown of conventional heterosexual family, not just by reassuring us that men are not obsolete in the reproduction process, but by keeping alternative family formations out of the frame—unless, like the homosexual couple in *The New Normal*, they conform to hetero-norms.[7] As Sarah Franklin (1990) argues, any forms of kinship outside of the traditional biological unit—adultery, single parents, illegitimacy, gay—is named and stigmatised as a 'lesser form of parenthood' (1990, 222). I argue that this is precisely what the narratives of these texts are doing by rendering alternative families invisible. They are also positioned as the losers in the story—as family outlaws. As Calhoun (2000) explains:

> At the same time that gay men and lesbians were publicly claiming to have genuine marriages and families of their own, it was becoming increasingly clear that heterosexuals were deviating in multiple ways from the conventional model of the two-parent, nuclear family. As in previous periods, constructing lesbians and gay men as dangerous outlaws to the family, diverting attention from heterosexuals' own choices to create multiple, new family arrangements that undermine the hegemony of the traditional family. In addition, the equation of heterosexuality with family values and homosexuality and lesbianism with hostility to the family serves to motivate loyalty to a traditional conception of the family. It also renders suspect some of the alternative family arrangements that heterosexuals might be inclined to choose, such as supportive, family-like relationships between women involved in single parenting. (2000, 153–154)

I believe this diversion is reflected in the texts, which also resonates with André Cavalcante's (2014) concept of anxious displacements, which is where excess anxiety is projected away from homosexual characters onto those in their orbit. I propose that through the postmodern family being situated outside of the representational frame, excess anxiety is being projected away from the conventional family unit, which is in decline, and onto any other alternative formations, situating them so far outside of the nuclear family frame that they disappear from view within mainstream popular culture. In relation to media and television images of the nuclear family, it has been argued that despite its decline, the normative nuclear family is fast-becoming a myth that needs to be reproduced and maintained—other formations made invisible—to be nostalgic, hopeful that the dominant social order will return (Burr and Jarvis 2007;

Naficy 1989; Tincknell 2005). As seen in the work of Halberstam (2011, 2013), this perpetuates the notion that despite its flaws, heteronormativity is still being articulated as the only game worth playing.

As highlighted in the previous chapter, ideologies of completeness, natural reproduction, romance, heterosexuality and whiteness have been identified in the analysis. However, in addition, and which will be central to the discussion here, is how the three focus groups (mixed mothers, non-mothers, and pre-mothers) have predominantly taken an oppositional position to the texts' narratives. I argue this is a form of resistance to the dominant discourses that have been identified.

What has also emerged, through the participants' discussion of love in relation to the attainment of a genetic child, is an eagerness to represent a wider range of creating families that do not *have* to be driven and created by genetic reproduction and the traditional family unit, but families that are created through more expansive notions of love. I argue that this is significant, as what has been identified in the audience data is a desire to embrace a counter-narrative of family, one which has been described by queer family scholars as fictive kin (Calhoun 2000)[8] and chosen families (Weston 1991).

Drawing on the participants' resistance to the core discourses in the texts, I argue that the cultural articulations of love and family in relation to the surrogacy storylines must be revised. Conventional family structures do not have to be positioned as aspirational for heterosexuals, homosexuals and lesbians to be deemed as respectable, moral citizens; and happy endings don't have to rely on the miracle of natural pregnancy or the building of family based on the genetic tie. It is also acceptable to portray positive female characters outside of motherhood.

Therefore, I propose that there is a desire for the dominant cultural space to articulate a more progressive, non-normative vision of family, alongside, but not necessarily instead of, the more traditional family unit, which as I have argued, has been constructed in the popular texts under analysis. I suggest, inspired by the research findings, that these alternative postmodern families can be built on a community of loved ones, not purely confined to the monogamous heterosexual couple dyad and the normative nuclear family unit, but built on a range of *connections* and alternative intimacies (Calhoun 2000; Halberstam 2011; Lehr 1999; Weston 1991). These 'chosen' families can include friends, lovers, couples, singles, mothers, non-mothers, gay, straight, genetic and non-genetic children, stepfamilies—even neighbours and animals

(Halberstam 2011). If anything, following Estella Tincknell (2005) it would be fair to propose that these new configurations of family do in fact have more value as they operate through cooperation outside of social expectations and familial obligation.

I argue this non-normative vision of family reflects more accurately the shift in kinship structures that exist in modern life, and which make valid, and normative, a range of identities for women (and men) which are not purely shaped through compulsory heterosexually.

I also propose that this research has revealed a space for a coalition politics between heterosexuality and homosexuality, categories that have tended to be so rigidly divided. Cathy Cohen (1997) has argued that heterosexuality should not be viewed as monolithic, and that heterosexuals can also feel marginalised by dominant ideologies of normative family and reproduction. While recognising that heterosexuality is a privileged identity position in comparison to homosexuality and lesbianism, I argue that the audience data supports this position.

Furthermore, through highlighting similarities, and by illuminating how oppressed subject positions of race, class, gender and sexuality have been made invisible, or subordinated, in the representations in focus, I propose that space must be made in the representational frame to include a range of kinship structures that are not solely focused on racial purity, and genetic bonds. I argue that the alternative intimacies that have emerged in queer and black culture would be helpful to draw upon for more varied cultural articulations of family, and that these kinship formations can transcend and dismantle the perpetuation of the myths and fantasies of normative family, which are embedded in these texts—narratives that imbue dominant ideologies of white classed privilege anchored in the preservation of the genetic tie.

Notes

1. Ien Ang has also explored the viewer displeasure of American soap operas. Ien Ang, *Watching Dallas: Soap Opera and the Melodramatic Imagination* (London: Routledge, 1985).
2. The childless female characters in TV dramas *Top of the Lake: China Girl* and *The Handmaid's Tale* also embody this narrative—they also long for a child more than their male partners. This is particularly distinct in *The Handmaid's Tale*, where The Commander's wife Serena is being consistently rejected by her husband. This has fueled her craving for a baby, as she wants 'a child to love'.

3. This is also illustrated in *Top of the Lake: China Girl* between lead character Robin and her estranged daughter Mary. Before they meet, Robin pines over a letter sent from a younger Mary. Their first meeting in a cafe signals a performance of a first date. When Mary, now 18, comes to Robin in distress, Robin holds her like a baby and sings to her. Robin gets a tattoo of her daughter's name on her wrist. This illustrates the love story between genetic mother and baby—but delayed due to separation.
4. HIV/Aids in predominantly heterosexual African communities has also impacted in a similar way within reshaping family, its victims also subjected to shame, stigmatisation and ejection from the family home (Epstein 2008).
5. Lugones and Rosezelle's (1995) debate on feminism and the term 'sisterhood' is a good example of what Rich (1979) has described as a white solipsism, which is the inability to relate to the non-white experience through an unconscious belief that one race is more superior over another.
6. The notion that gay men are harmful to children is still being perpetuated in contemporary cinema, as seen in *Ideal Home* (2018). Despite being based on the personal experiences of the director Andrew Fleming, the two leading gay characters (played by eminent straight actors Steve Coogan and Paul Rudd) are still shaped by these stereotypes. They are portrayed as emotionally immature and a potential danger to children through an obsession with porn, drug and alcohol use and dangerous driving. The characteristics of the 'swishy effeminate queen' (Walters 2001, 61) which have been used to paint gay characters since the 1960s is also evident.
7. Also see Hamid Naficy's (1989) discussion on how the family myth 'percolates through TV texts' despite acknowledging the changes in its normative structure. Naficy argues this percolation 'does not question the basic institution of family itself and the monogamous heterosexual coupling which it entails'. Naficy, "Television Intertextuality," 49.
8. The concept of 'fictive kin' is an anthropological term, which has been used to describe kin that has historically been viewed as not real, due to not having a blood connection, such as a godparent or adopted child. Weston (1991) proposes that although the concept lost popularity in the social sciences, it has become a valid and useful term by which to describe the gay communities who have chosen their families, especially due to mainstream society's resistance to accept these new formations as authentic and as valuable. This has been identified through how the media articulate these kinship bonds, using phrases such as 'pretended family relations' and 'so-called family' which are 'recurrently applied to lesbian or gay couples, parents, and families of friends' (Weston 1991, 106).

References

Ahmed, Sara. 2006. *Queer Phenomenology: Orientations, Objects, Others*. London: Routledge.

Ahmed, Sara. 2010. *The Promise of Happiness*. Durham: Duke University Press.

Ang, Ien. 1985. *Watching Dallas: Soap Opera and the Melodramatic Imagination*. New ed. London: Routledge.

Ang, Ien. 1995. *Living Room Wars*. London: Routledge.

Arnold, Emily A., and Marlon M. Bailey. 2009. "Constructing Home and Family: How the Ballroom Community Supports Africa American GLBTQ Youth in the Face of HIV/AIDS." *Journal of Gay and Lesbian Social Services* 21 (2–3): 171–188.

Barrett, Michèle, and Mary McIntosh. 1991. *The Anti-social Family*. New York: Verso.

Barry, Kathleen. 1985. *Female Sexual Slavery*. New York: New York University Press.

Berlant, Lauren. 1994. "America, 'Fat,' the Fetus'." *Boundary 2* 21 (3): 145–195.

Berlant, Lauren. 2008. *The Female Complaint*. Durham: Duke University Press.

Birke, Lynda, and Joanna Hockenhull. 2012. *Crossing Boundaries: Investigating Human-Animal Relationships*. Boston: Brill.

Birke, Lynda, and Joanna Hockenhull. 2016. "Moving With(in) Affect. Horses, People and Tolerance." In *Affect, Space, and Animals*, edited by Jopi Nyman and Nora Schuurman. Abingdon: Routledge.

Briggs, Laura. 2017. *How All Politics Became Reproductive Politics—From Welfare Reform to Foreclosure to Trump*. Berkeley: University of California Press.

Browne, Kath, and Catherine Nash. 2010. *Queer Methods and Methodologies: Intersecting Queer Theories and Social Science Research*. New York: Routledge.

Burr, Vivienne, and Christine Jarvis. 2007. "Imagining the Family: Representations of Alternative Lifestyles in Buffy the Vampire Slayer." *Qualitative Social Work* 6 (3): 263–280.

Butler, Judith. 1993. *Bodies That Matter: On the Discursive Limits of Sex*. London: Routledge.

Calhoun, Cheshire. 2000. *Feminism, Family, and the Politics of the Closet: Lesbian and Gay Displacement*. Oxford: Oxford University Press.

Carsten, Janet. 2004. *After Kinship*. Cambridge: Cambridge University Press.

Cavalcante, André. 2014. "Anxious Displacements: The Representation of Gay Parenting on Modern Family and The New Normal and the Management of Cultural Anxiety." *Television & New Media* 1 (18): 454–471.

Charles, Nickie. 2014. "Post-Human Families? Dog-Human Relations in the Domestic Sphere." *Sociological Research Online* 21 (3): 715–730.

Charles, Nickie. 2016. "'Animals Just Love You as You Are': Experiencing Kinship Across the Species Barrier." *Sociology* 48 (4): 715–730.
Charles, Nickie, and Charlotte Aull Davies. 2008. "My Family and Other Animals: Pets as Kin." *Sociological Research Online* 13 (5).
Chauncey, George. 1995. *Gay New York: Gender, Urban Culture, and the Making of the Gay Male World, 1890–1940.* New York: Basic Books.
Cohen, Cathy J. 1997. "Punks, Bulldaggers, and Welfare Queens: The Radical Potential of Queer Politics?" *GLQ: A Journal of Lesbian and Gay Studies* 3 (4): 437–465.
Demory, Pamela, and Christopher Pullen. 2013. *Queer Love in Film and Television.* New York: Palgrave Macmillan.
Edelman, Lee. 2003. *No Future: Queer Theory and the Death Drive.* Durham: Duke University Press.
Epstein, Helen. 2008. *The Invisible Cure: Africa, the West and the Fight Against AIDS.* London: Penguin.
Evans, Mary. 2003. *Love: An Unromantic Discussion.* Cambridge: Polity Press.
Firestone, Shulamith. 1970. *Dialectic of Sex: The Case for a Feminist Revolution.* New York: Naomi Wolf.
Fiske, John. 1989. *Reading the Popular.* London: Routledge.
Folger, Tom. 2008. "Queer Nuclear Families? Reproducing and Transgressing Heteronormativity." *Journal of Homosexuality* 54 (1–2): 124–149. http://dx.doi.org/10.1080/00918360801952028.
Franklin, Sarah. 1990. "Deconstructing Desperateness': The Social Construction of Infertility in Popular Representations of New Reproductive Technologies" In *The New Reproductive Technologies*, edited by Maureen McNeil. London: Palgrave Macmillan.
Fudge, Erica. 2008. *Pets (The Art of Living).* London: Routledge.
Gorton, Kristyn. 2009. *Media Audiences.* Edinburgh: Edinburgh University Press.
Halberstam, Judith. 2011. *The Queer Art of Failure.* Durham: Duke University Press.
Halberstam, Judith. 2013. *Gaga Feminism: Sex, Gender and the End of Normal.* Boston: Beacon Press.
Halbert, Deborah. 2004. "Shulamith Firestone." *Information, Communication & Society* 7 (1):115–135. https://doi.org/10.1080/1369118042000208933.
Haraway, Donna. 2007. *When Species Meet.* Minneapolis: University of Minnesota Press.
Klepfisz, Irena. 1999. "It Is Not a Child I Wish to Mother, It Is Myself." *Reproductive Health Matters* 7 (13): 96–102.
Lam, Carla. 2015. *New Reproductive Technologies and Disembodiment.* 1st ed. Abingdon: Routledge.

Lehr, Valerie. 1999. *Queer Family Values: Debunking the Myth of the Nuclear Family*. Philadelphia: Temple University Press.

Lugones, Maria, and Pat Rosezelle. 1995. "Sisterhood and Friendship as Feminist Models." In *Feminism and Community*, edited by Penny Weiss and Marilyn Friedman. Philadelphia: Temple University Press.

MacDowell, James. 2013. *Happy Endings in Hollywood Cinema: Cliché, Convention and the Final Couple*. Edinburgh: Edinburgh University Press.

Merck, Mandy, and Stella Sandford. 2010. *Further Adventures of the Dialectic of Sex*. 1st ed. New York: Palgrave Macmillan.

Miller, Tina. 2005. *Making Sense of Motherhood: A Narrative Approach*. Cambridge: Cambridge University Press.

Naficy, Hamid. 1989. "Television Intertextuality and the Discourse of the Nuclear Family." *Journal of Film and Video* 41 (4): 42–59.

Oliver, Kelly. 2012. *Knock Me Up, Knock Me Down*. New York: Columbia University Press.

Park, Shelley. 2014. *Mothering Queerly, Queering Motherhood*. New York: State University of New York Press.

Radway, Janice. 1983. "Women Read the Romance: The Interaction of Text and Context." *Feminist Studies* 9 (1): 53–78.

Radway, Janice. 1992. *Reading the Romance: Women, Patriarchy, and Popular Literature*. 2nd ed. Chapel Hill, NC: University North Carolina.

Rich, Adrienne. 1979. "'Disloyal to Civilization': Feminism, Racism, and Gynephobia." *Chrysalis* 7: 9–27.

Rich, Adrienne. 1980. "Compulsory Heterosexuality and Lesbian Existence." *Signs: Journal of Women in Culture and Society* 5 (4): 631–660.

Roberts, Dorothy. 1995. "The Genetic Tie." *The University of Chicago Law Review* 62 (1): 209–273.

Roberts, Dorothy. 1996. "Race and the New Reproduction." *Faculty Scholarship at Penn Law*. 1154.

Rubin, Lilian. 1993. *Just Friends: The Role of Friendship in Our Lives*. New York: Harper Perennial.

Schlichter, Annette. 2004. "Queer at Last? Straight Intellectuals and the Desire for Transgression." *GLQ: A Journal of Lesbian and Gay Studies* 10 (4): 543–564.

Skeggs, Beverley, and Helen Wood. 2008. "The Labour of Transformation and Circuits 'Around' Reality Television." *Continuum: Journal of Media & Cultural Studies* 22 (4): 559–572.

Smart, Carol. 2011. "Ways of Knowing: Crossing Species Boundaries." *Methodological Innovations*, 6 (3): 27–38.

Stacey, Jackie. 1993. *Star Gazing: Hollywood Cinema and Female Spectatorship*. 1st ed. New York: Routledge.

Tincknell, Estella. 2005. *Mediating the Family: Gender, Culture and Representation*. London: Bloomsbury.

Waitress. 2007. Directed and Written by Adrien Shelly. Film. Los Angeles, CA: Fox.

Walters, Suzanna. 1996. "From Here to Queer: Radical Feminism, Postmodernism, and the Lesbian Menace (or, Why Can't a Woman Be More Like a Fag?)." *Signs* 21 (4): 830–869.

Walters, Suzanna. 2001. *All the Rage: The Story of Gay Visibility in America*. Chicago: University of Chicago Press.

Warner, Michael. 1999. *The Trouble with Normal*. Cambridge, MA: Harvard University Press.

Weston, Kath. 1991. *Families We Choose*. 1st ed. New York: Columbia University Press.

What to Expect When You're Expecting. 2012. Directed by Kirk Jones. Written by Shauna Cross, Heather Hach, Heidi Murkoff. Film. Santa Monica, CA: Lionsgate.

CHAPTER 6

Conclusion: Why Representation on TV Matters

Picture Imperfect

The initial aim of this study was to explore how the participants made sense of the practice of surrogacy through its representation on popular platforms of TV and film. One of the central research questions selected to support this aim asked what the narratives of surrogacy in the shows selected for analysis represent in relation to conventional notions of motherhood and family. The findings presented in Chapter 2 offer some enlightening responses to this. Focusing on two texts, *Giuliana & Bill* and *Coronation Street*, the participants discussed how the surrogates and the intended mothers were positioned in the visual frame (on the screen), how they were constructed as characters within the narrative, and what this implied in regard to the imbalance of power between them. In the context of this chapter, this was recognised through how the surrogate Delphine in *Giuliana & Bill* was represented, with the participants stating that her lack of physical voice and increasing disappearance off the screen inferred quite unashamedly that she was being positioned as subordinate to the intended mother, Giuliana.

Through the participants being able to acknowledge the disparities of privilege and power between the two characters due to how they were portrayed, a specific type of user of reproductive technologies was identified—white, coupled, heterosexual and middle class. This is significant as this specific type presented in the texts is also reflected in the ideal

L. Le Vay, *Surrogacy and the Reproduction of Normative Family on TV*, Palgrave Studies in Science and Popular Culture,
https://doi.org/10.1007/978-3-030-17570-2_6

category of the user that is constructed through media and medical discourses of infertility. By identifying this ideal user, it was argued that subjects positioned outside of this constructed ideal were marginalised from dominant representation through race, social class, sexual orientation and marital status. The audience data showed that the surrogate Delphine was underrepresented in the narrative, and on the screen. Therefore, I was able to conclude through textual analysis that an inclusion in the frame would disturb the norms of conventional family that the texts were aiming to reinforce. It can also be proposed that such norms also drive the reproductive technologies agenda, despite notions that technologies, when embraced by same-sex parents, are able to bend norms by creating new formations of family. This was identified through the participants recognising how the representations worked to attach value to the genetic connection, heteronormative (and homonormative) monogamy and women's role in reproduction, either through adopting a maternal identity (as the intended mother) or through assisting the production of a child (the surrogate). The ideology of racial purity, although indistinctly pointed to through the audience data, was identified primarily through textual analysis.

Furthermore, the complexities of engaging with reproductive technologies that arose in the discussions between the participants also emerged as noteworthy, explicitly in relation to the wider implications of the pressures put on women's reproductive obligations that they were unsettled by. The main difficulty that was identified in the texts by the participants was the lack of alternative choices outside of motherhood represented to mainstream television audiences, which became a dominant theme throughout the project. Despite the participants showing an understanding of the transformative disciplinary power of reproductive technologies, the fundamental message they pinpointed—that they understood as being core to these two texts, and throughout all of the texts in focus—is that the goal of the narrative for the female characters is to get the baby, no matter what, 'by hook or by crook' (Sonja, mixed mothers focus group). However, as they highlighted, this was conditional on the female subject being of a privileged status, which allows them access to reproductive technologies.

As was identified by both participants and the textual analysis, this privileged status was predominantly white, heterosexual and middle class. This therefore helped precede the primary conclusion in this chapter that certain classed, sexually orientated and raced bodies are excluded from representation, situated outside of normative white heterosexual culture which steers the narratives, positioning them as deviant, non-normative. This finding is important as such representations illuminate which bodies are considered culturally compatible with motherhood and family, and which are not, which as aforementioned also reflects the central beliefs inferred through medical discourses. As Sarah Franklin (1990) proposes: 'popular representations are a powerful force in the social world and cultural construction of reproduction' (1990, 227).

Race in relation to reproductive technologies has also emerged as of core importance in this book. Scholars in this field, particularly Dorothy Roberts (1995, 1996, 2000), have explored the way images of the practice are constructed and mediated to denote white privilege through policies and news stories, which Roberts has argued is symbolic of the preservation of the genetic tie, which signifies the importance of racial purity. The genetic tie in relation to acquiring a child—through surrogacy or natural pregnancy—is also a core theme that has been identified as significant throughout this book. I believe the discussion of how certain bodies are excluded from the representational frame, alongside how black bodies are articulated within the texts—in relation to reproductive technologies, maternal abilities and the support of white happiness—has engaged with and developed Roberts' work. As Roberts highlights in her discussion of the genetic tie as a social import, which I believe deeply resonates with core themes of race within this work:

> The genetic tie plays a role in constructing several dimensions of identity; it helps to define that person, the family, and the nation. It may inspire an intimate bond between a parent and a child, as well as constitute a legislated prerequisite for inclusion in an entire race of people. (1995, 211)

Like Roberts, and to some extent, Kelly Oliver (2012), who has explored representations of race and pregnancy in Hollywood films, I too have been able to identify and discuss racial subtexts, but through exploring contemporary texts, and their reception, with a specific focus on surrogacy. Furthermore, Roberts' proposition that a more alternative vision of family is possible outside of the genetic tie, inspired by black communities, has also been engaged with inspired by the research findings—to be discussed further on.

I Feel for You

Two of the central research questions asked how, and if, narratives of surrogacy are articulated differently due to the varying techniques of each genre, and what impact these techniques may have had on how the participants understood the practice. The texts that were selected for the focus group viewing sessions included sitcom, documentary, drama, Hollywood mom-com, reality TV and soap opera—a wide range of genres specifically chosen for this purpose. Initially, documentary and drama were excluded. This was decided upon to narrow the focus for the book, analytical attention paid to not only more popular mainstream texts, but to those texts with stronger surrogacy storylines. However, as explained in the introductory chapter, two key TV dramas materialised after the ethnographic research was undertaken—*Top of the Lake: China Girl and The Handmaid's Tale*. These shows will be explored in relation to this book's findings further on and will be revisited in a separate, more in-depth research project. These shows are important and deserve close analysis, which cannot be dealt with here. After all, who knows what narratives might emerge in the subsequent series of *The Handmaid's Tale*?

Although documentary was also excluded, the findings that were garnered from the research process were certainly not wasted, as many aspects of its filming techniques were utilised for the genre analysis component of this project. This was valuable, as it materialised that its core formulae influenced the body of work in focus, specifically *The New Normal*. Participants detected the appearance of what looked like the use of a hand-held camera 'zooming around' (Rose, pre-mothers focus group), a technique of cinema verité that is intended to create a fly-on-the-wall perspective.

What surfaced as meaningful in the audience data was how effective the genre techniques actually were in evoking emotional responses from the viewers, particularly by enabling a connection with the main characters. It was interesting to establish which genre techniques were successful in generating emotional and empathetic responses from the participants, and which weren't, in relation to how the different genres constructed emotions in the texts. This was established by analysing the narrative building of shots, sequences of scenes, camera work, acting style, positioning of characters, dialogue and close-up shots. Through this analysis what emerged as significant was how this worked—or how it didn't work—on the viewers. As Noël Carroll (1996) emphasises:

'Through critical prefocusing we could say that the filmmaker leads the horse to water. But the circuit is not completed until the audience drinks' (in Gorton 2009, 79).

During the discussion of *Rules of Engagement* and *Giuliana & Bill*, participants showed they were much more able to relate to the emotions expressed by the leading female infertile character Audrey in *Rules of Engagement*, through 'emotional stimulation' (Smith 1995, 97) than with Giuliana in *Giuliana & Bill*. This is where the viewers are able to project themselves into the scene and empathise with the character's situation. Although both of these shows were the least liked by viewers, *Giuliana & Bill* was the most disliked—the participants viewed the couple as narcissistic, and the production of the show insincere and distasteful. This therefore indicates a failure of the construction of emotional stimulation in the text. Although this is a reality TV genre, it did not paint an empathetic picture of surrogacy to the participants, primarily due to what they believed was a disrespectful under-representation of the surrogate, as discussed in the previous section. It was not just how she is physically positioned on the screen/within the frame, but through a distinct lack of vocal presence. In short: the audience refused to drink the water.

In contrast, *Coronation Street* aroused the most compassion and understanding of the surrogacy practice out of all of the texts that were viewed, particularly being able to empathise with the childless character, Izzy. The focus group participants identified key genre differences between the shows and formed more meaningful emotional connections with the text through how the genre techniques articulated the practice. This emerged through how the narrative structuring and characterisations were able to communicate the complexities of surrogacy, principally by identifying the maternal power struggle between the two women—the surrogate (the birth mother) and the intended mother (the genetic mother). It has been identified that this maternal tension in the narrative acts as a mechanism by which to create voids between women. Such friction has been read a concern, therefore a discussion about how these characters are formed and interact are to follow. Furthermore, the participants believed *Giuliana & Bill*—as a show and as characters—to be insincere, fake and at times nauseating to watch, 'like eating a bag of sweets' (Carla, mixed mothers focus group). In contrast, *Coronation Street* was thought of as more sensitive to the issues, by not only showing multiple viewpoints of the characters involved, which is one of soap opera's central genre devices, but also through how information on the practice was incorporated into the narrative through the scripting. As explained by Rebecca (non-mothers focus group): 'You got the most information about it all – the procedures *and* the feelings and emotions'.

A key finding, therefore, is that soap opera's techniques of executing the surrogacy narrative was the most successful in being able to encourage the participants to be the most sensitive and empathetic to a representation of the practice, despite the TV show being fictional. This was primarily due to the way empathy for the characters is shaped through its narrative devices of exploring emotionally complex issues through multiple viewpoints, which are able to engage audiences through the structure of sympathy. Furthermore, it can be argued that this affective engagement with the characters is also the result of the serial form of the soap opera—where characters are shaped over longer periods of time—the melodramatic women-centred direction of the genre which magnifies the disruptions and resolutions of the storylines, which keep the viewers hooked, and the reflection of elements of real life, that can be complex.

Although all of these genre elements can also be identified in the production of *Giuliana & Bill*, the impact was not as fruitful. It can be suggested that this is due to the characters having already been recognised as celebrities prior to the show, with the narrative focus purely on them, and not the surrogate, and the differences in the production of the show due to it being a more 'docusoap' style of reality TV show, which prioritises entertainment value over more meaningful social issues (Bruzzi 2001). For example, the hosting network E! is a celebrity and entertainment news channel which flags up its other entertainment shows during airing. It was this, specifically, that some of the participants thought was distasteful in relation to the practice of commercial surrogacy deserving a more sensitive representation.

Playing It Straight

A key research question asks what the narratives of surrogacy represent in relation to notions of not just motherhood, but family. It has been identified that narratives in all of the texts revolve around a central notion that a couple must have children, ideally genetically related to at least one parent, to complete their family—to be considered a *real* family. As Sonja (mixed mothers focus group, 2015) emphasised: 'It's not a gay or straight thing – the concept of family not being a family unless there are children involved'. What Sonja highlighted, which materialised as a core finding in the research, is that conventional notions of family are also embedded in the central narratives of *The New Normal* and *Rules of Engagement*, which feature homosexual and lesbian characters. Also, to some extent, in *Baby Mama*, due to the lesbian connotations between the intended mother and the surrogate.

It emerged in the audience data that representations of homosexual men, such as characters Bryan and David in *The New Normal*, must be seen to express a desire for a genetic child, within a monogamous relationship, to be viewed as normal. As Jackie (mixed mothers focus group, 2015) pointed out: 'it makes them more acceptable'. Through this recognition of how same-sex relationships are normalised in the narrative, it was argued that to become normal, to be ordinary, was a desire that had to be exhibited by a homosexual to be able to assimilate into the mainstream, to be part of an acceptable community—to be tolerated. *Queer straightness* was a concept I introduced and applied to the analysis to describe this process of straightening. Extending Sara Ahmed's (2010) work on straightening devices, which defines how certain scripts of happiness are used to align bodies within compulsory heterosexuality, *queer straightness* illustrates a direction, or a set of behaviours and living practices, which homosexuals must embrace to avoid being considered unnatural.

The key conclusion here was that the notion of homosexuality as a lifestyle—sexual practice removed from view, to be discussed below—is only tolerable if presented as showing an allegiance to the family ideal: two parents, romantic love, a genetic child and a family home. I believe this to be a poignant revelation that has been identified in the data—a process of normalisation that doesn't challenge straight culture but mirrors it—the primary aim to placate social anxieties of homosexuality (and lesbianism) under certain terms. As has been revealed through this book, for LGBTQ television representations to be accepted into the mainstream the character constructions and the narratives within which they reside must adhere to the heteronormative—to traditional notions of family. In short, queers must behave to make it onto primetime television and film. As Michael Warner (1999) highlights in relation to heterosexual dominance and media representations, but which can now be applied to these more contemporary cultural articulations of homosexuality and family:

> People are constantly encouraged to believe that heterosexual desire, dating, marriage, reproduction, childrearing, and home life are not only valuable to themselves, but the bedrock on which every other value in the world rests. Heterosexual desire and romance are thought to be the very core of humanity... It is the one thing celebrated in every film plot, every sitcom, every advertisement. (1999, 47)

While it is important to acknowledge the argument that such representations might challenge, or destabilise, conventional ideals of family, by exhibiting a resistance to dominant norms, they are problematic as such narratives reproduce norms and mainstream values. For example, the final equilibrium of *The New Normal* mirrors the endings of the other texts under analysis. This idea of the sexual disciplining of gay characters to enable reproduction was also identified in the representation of the lesbian surrogate, Brenda, in *Rules of Engagement.* By becoming a surrogate Brenda is removed from a lesbian relationship and relocated into the heterosexual couple's home, where she is monitored during her pregnancy. The couple acquires the genetic child that they were so desperate for, to become a *real* family—happy, complete. Therefore, despite bending norms by inserting gay characters into conventional family structures, the norms flex back into a similar shape, although slightly distorted. Furthermore, what has also surfaced as noteworthy in relation to this idea of straightening gay characters to make them more acceptable, primarily to mainstream heterosexual audiences, was that to do so, sexual intimacy between same-sex couples has to be eradicated, disciplined, through the notion of monogamy, domesticity and romantic love, which is placed at the forefront of the narrative. Sexual intimacy is obscured to pave the way for the child. This is a concealment, which I believe can only be aided by the separation of sex from reproduction. Gay visibility is therefore only tolerated as long as it is acknowledged as an identity, and not performed as a sexual act.

It was also proposed that this normative shape, created by impressions of heteronormativity (Ahmed 2006) had been formed through how the homosexual characters have been constructed in relation to normative notions of parenthood and family. I decided one way to explore this was through detecting traces of the lesbian concept of butch/femme in the construction of the homosexual characters. Through this pairing, it was argued that conventional gender roles were adhered to (masculine/feminine, man/woman, father/mother) to make same-sex parenting more palatable to mainstream audiences. Employing butch/femme as a flexible concept worked as an analytical lens, as the masculine/feminine roles in relation to the construction of same-sex couples also re-emerge in the ambiguous relationship between the two women in *Baby Mama*. This performance of masculine/feminine traits which surface through the father/father and mother/mother roles have been drawn from a 'masculinization of motherhood' (Lam 2015, 33) inspired by Paula's (non-mothers focus group, 2015) response to all of the representations of the intended mothers in the texts: 'They [the intended mothers] must feel the way a father must feel'. This statement describes anxieties in relation to maternal identity and position within the traditional parental frame and refers to how the genetic mother has been removed from the gestational process. This statement materialised as particularly poignant throughout the book, as it clearly signifies a shift in the maternal role, and therefore, as argued, also creates a space to reassign gender traits, as seen in the performances of gender in the texts.

A main finding in relation to the changeability of gender traits, which was established as important to the participants, was how the use of the stereotype in the sitcom genre is employed to reinforce notions of femininity in relation to pregnancy and motherhood. Where it was supposed that femininity and masculinity are performed through the butch/femme model to make homosexual parenting and coupling in *The New Normal* more digestible to mainstream audiences, a similar manipulation of character gender traits were also noted by the participants as important, particularly in relation to Brenda, the lesbian surrogate in *Rules of Engagement*. Brenda's shift from being portrayed as unwomanly to womanly, from masculine to feminine, through the pregnancy process was also argued to be a device by which to placate mainstream audience's anxieties of the disruption of normative reproductive processes.

Through the participants recognising how the stereotype works in the portrayal of lesbianism (and homosexuality) I was able to identify how conventional notions of femininity in relation to pregnancy and motherhood are reinforced, which I argued points to how heterosexist ideologies are embedded in the texts. This feminising, or as I have named them, drawing on Ahmed (2010), this *straightening* of the masculine lesbian through pregnancy provoked negative responses from many of the participants, regardless of their sexual orientation. However, it was the bisexual participant Jackie (mixed mothers focus group), who expressed how she thought the inclusion of lesbian (and homosexual) characters is better than no representation at all—and does in fact indicate an advance. Disappointingly, this echoes similar responses to compromises of lesbian representations made by writers of lesbian novels in the 1950s, such as *Spring Fire* (1952) author Vin Packer. This reflects feminist film theorists' beliefs that the narrative closure may be less important than making visible marginalised lives.

Although this idea of compromise in relation to lesbian representation warrants further exploration through audience research, to be discussed further on, what is important to focus on here in the context of this work is how lesbians are represented as culturally incompatible with motherhood. Brenda in *Rules of Engagement* is shown as having no interest in becoming a mother to her own genetic child or wanting to keep the baby she is carrying for someone else. Kate and Angie in *Baby Mama* do not form a lesbian relationship and become same-sex parents to a child. The final equilibrium in the narrative is that they have their own genetic babies through normative heterosexual relationships, whether they remain coupled or not (the surrogate Angie splits from her partner but he remains in the parental picture). Through the initial search for texts that feature surrogacy storylines only the hit American medical drama *Grey's Anatomy* has a brief lesbian couple surrogacy storyline (Season 10, Episode 24: 'Fear [Of the Unknown]') which ends up with the couple divorcing (and no baby). This was not selected for focus group viewing as the drama genre was removed for focus. These representations show how ideological dominant notions of femininity are repeated. The findings in this book illustrate how the female-only audiences have resisted the dominant heterosexist encodings in the text's narratives in relation to lesbian (and homosexual) representations *and* representations of heterosexual female infertility.

All Woman

A poignant finding that emerged through the research was how the participants not only rejected notions of femininity that are shaped in the texts, in relation to norms of motherhood and heterosexual coupling, but were also irritated by how the childless characters are positioned within the narrative. Focusing primarily on two key texts, *Baby Mama* and *Rules of Engagement*, the annoyance felt by viewers was that to be considered a real and complete woman, one has to become a mother, situated within a heterosexual couple dyad. Laura (non-mothers focus group) believed the texts were trying to say: 'You're not a real woman until you've had a child'. It was clear that for many of the participants that the necessity for the narratives to conclude in natural pregnancies, or in the acquisition of a genetic child through surrogacy, was exclusionary to other feminine identities. The defaulting to a normative image of family was also regarded as 'a cop out' (Jackie, mixed mothers focus group). This was due to the narrative not allowing space to explore more alternative endings. As pointed out by Carrie (same group): 'It's as if people can't quite cope with the idea of women who can't have children'.

What emerged as significant was how some of the participants were able to discuss their own experiences of feeling alienated and positioned as non-normative in their everyday lives, in relation to normative feminine ideals of motherhood and family, when discussing how the stories concluded. This was most revealing in relation to the key research question, which asked how the representations of motherhood reflected women's own situated experiences of living in the world. Sally's (mixed mothers focus group) openness about her own experiences as a single and childless heterosexual woman, in particular, illuminated how heterosexual romance and specific notions of heteronormative motherhood are central to shaping some women's life narratives—as this research has revealed is evident both on and off screen. Just as the characters in the texts evoked social anxieties that needed to be placated with normative solutions, Sally also shared how during social engagements she would often be grilled about her identity as a woman in relation to motherhood and a monogamous heterosexual relationship, as if these attributes were seen as necessary for having social value and a primary requisite of femininity. Recounting a social event, she said: 'I was like, "hello! You know, actually my name is Sally, and would you like to learn something about me rather than these add-ons?"' In this statement Sally was describing herself as *already* whole and completed, anything outside of her already shaped identity was an added extra, which conflicts with the ideology of completeness which underpins all of the texts' narratives. Most importantly, these findings reveal how such notions of what it means to be a woman, which are shaped through the heterosexual romance narrative, are myths; myths which are prolific throughout popular culture. What has been identified in this book is that these myths are still being perpetuated through the characterisation and narrative construction in these contemporary texts. Like the non-mothers portrayed in the stories, Sally also felt she was being positioned on the outside of social norms.

Although the participants read the childless female characters as heterosexual—and read the clearly signed lesbian characters as lesbian—a correlation between how these characters are constructed and the lesbian subject position was drawn. This was due to identifying similarities between the two subject positions through how they both disturb the category 'woman', by being seen as incomplete. As I argued, the lesbian is also viewed as non-normative—seen as a failure to become a real woman, and a threat to heterosexual reproduction. Although this comparison was a risky approach to take, I believe it was an important one to make. My aim was to make it transparent in the discussion and analysis of the findings that the parallels drawn between the two positions in no way detract from the far more serious exclusionary practices (access to reproductive technologies, parental legal status, cultural representations) which have, and still do, face lesbian women in modern life. This comparison was inspired through the participants' discussion of how the intended mothers on the screen are removed from the gestational process, which positions them as fathers. This created the narrative space for sexual identities and gender roles to perform more ambiguously in the texts, particularly seen in the portrayal of the two women in *Baby Mama*, which played with lesbian connotation. The core of the film's narrative focussed on the pair sharing a domestic space and the expectation of a child—despite the surrogate's pregnancy initially being faked—with no stable male partners present. Therefore, a queer reading open to possible erotic nuances in texts was deemed necessary, primarily by my own textual analysis in dialogue with the participants' responses, to unearth any heterosexist ideologies embedded in the text.

The analysis was able to reveal how all sexual ambiguities *and* infertility are erased through how the stories concluded—heterosexual romance, natural pregnancy. Drawing parallels between lesbian sexual identity and heterosexual infertility adds richness to the findings and offers a progressive contribution to the field of queer media theory. However, I also recognise that this proposition should also be viewed as the instigator of a conversation that can, and should, be developed further, continuing to expand the use of the term *queer*, and to use it as a device to describe those who fail to comply to norms, which, as has been outlined, includes subject positions on both sides of the hetero/homo binary. This notion of failing to conform to norms chimes with Judith Halberstam's (2011) work on queerness and failure. Halberstam (2011) argues that the winners in the story are always the white nuclear families—lesbians and homosexuals situated as the losers, the failures. To be represented as incomplete—in this discussion, as a lesbian or childless heterosexual woman, as depicted in the representations under analysis—signifies loss, unhappiness. However, as Halberstam points out, there is strength in failing, in losing. Through failure she believes new possibilities open up—new pathways. Interestingly, this stance is reflected in Karen Throsby's (2004) qualitative work on IVF failure, where it was only after some of the women in her sample stopped IVF that confidence was regained, and prosperous new beginnings blossomed, primarily in being able to pursue and actualise their career ambitions.

Furthermore, the ideology of completeness—that a woman is not viewed as complete until she has become a mother—also resonates with how reproductive technologies function through a disciplinary power (Farquhar 1996; Foucault 1977). As discussed earlier in this chapter, it has been proposed that disciplinary power has the potential to have a transformative effect on the body, that is both 'liberatory and controlling' (Farquhar 1996, 6). Controlling in the sense that, as described by Sonja (mixed mothers focus group) reproductive technologies puts additional pressure on women to reproduce and unshackling in the sense that science has yielded many different options to consider. The participants recognised that the representation of surrogacy in the narratives performed as a vehicle by which to enable the infertile female characters to become mothers by obtaining a genetic baby born through surrogacy. Any other lifestyle choices, such as deciding to not have children/become a mother, were blocked. All of these female characters were portrayed as desperately wanting to have a genetic child, and were able, through the narrative, to use reproductive technologies to assist them. They were also able to have access to another woman's body to gestate their genetic child, to facilitate their maternal desire.

As the participants detected, the worst thing that could happen in these stories was for the female characters to 'not get the baby' (Carla, mixed mothers focus group), which would position them as failures by not conforming to feminine ideals, particularly if they chose a career over motherhood (Oliver 2012). It was this obsessive drive to become a mother through any means possible that disturbed the participants the most. The audience data revealed that a heterosexual woman could not be imagined as anything other than a mother, domesticated and settled within a normative family unit—restored to a normative female position (Kuhn 1992). 'Normal service', as Sonja described, had to be resumed at the end of every narrative. It was these dominant encodings in the texts that the participants rejected, as many felt that they would like to see different endings that are less conventional, with the female protagonists not getting the baby as the narrative conclusion. As Laura (non-mothers focus group) stated: 'It's great that these fictional characters can get pregnant, but it's kind of a shame that it can't be left as you can't have kids, you know what I mean?... It would be interesting if someone wrote that into a story instead of doing the nice Hollywood ending'.

For the characters, it isn't just heterosexual love that rescues them from their infertility, but reproductive technologies also. 'By hook, or by crook' for the stories to be complete, the heterosexual women have to become mothers, which, as it emerged, is a desire that eclipses the romance narrative. In these stories, having a baby and becoming a mother is the dominant desire—more important than getting (or keeping) the man. As Rhian (pre-mothers focus group) pinpointed in her response to *Baby Mama*: 'There was no love at first, but she wanted a child to love... otherwise your life is pointless'. Moreover, I argue one of the most significant aspects of this research project is how childless heterosexual women are pictured as a reproductive threat to the future, which as pointed out by Carrie (mixed mothers focus group) is a core anxiety that shapes the narratives in all of the texts, one which she claims assumes that audiences would find it difficult to accept.

We Are Family

The participants oppositional reading of the majority of the texts under analysis is revealing in the sense that it exposed that a range of women, from a variety of different positions on motherhood, want to see different endings with a more progressive narrative shape to a woman's life, in relation to the normative path of motherhood and family. It was recognised by the participants that a woman's happiness and fulfilment should not be solely wrapped up in obtaining the happy object (Ahmed 2010) of the genetic child to become a mother. The participants also believed that alternative life paths should be made visible, positively, rather than portraying childless women as failures, and not wholly feminine, which is what these texts suggest. As Laura (non-mothers focus group) argued:

> It's not necessarily a sad ending if they [the intended mothers] can't have children, because we knew that from the beginning that they couldn't. If

> they have a child through surrogacy, they've got a child. It doesn't mean they have to get pregnant by natural means to conclude the story, to complete her as a person and as a woman.
>
> (Laura, non-mothers focus group, 2015)

It was also felt by the participants that the emphasis was more on the characters' desire to transform into the mother identity through the acquisition of a child, rather than on the child itself. This was interpreted by some participants as selfish, and only enabled through a position of privilege—those who could afford to access reproductive technologies. This was particularly evident in the discussion of *Giuliana & Bill*, where it was felt that the baby was simply another object that was purchased to show off to the cameras.

A key finding in the research, in response to how the narratives in all of the texts under analysis are driven by the desire to acquire a genetic child, was the debunking of the myth of the love-at-first-sight mother–child bond. As I have argued, the drive to become a mother by acquiring a genetic child has displaced the romantic love narrative from central focus—the search for love, and the romantic notion of falling in love, is now attached to the baby, rather than the man. It emerged as significant that Carrie and Sonja, the mothers in the focus groups, were not able to relate to the notion of the instant love bond with the child at birth, and even throughout motherhood later on. They believed their experiences of motherhood were not reflected in the representations. They too felt excluded, similarly to Sally (mixed mothers focus group) who, due to being single and childless, explained how she felt positioned outside of dominant norms. Both Sonja and Carrie believed that maternal love is changeable—not instant or even presumed—but an affection that grows slowly over time. The mothers also expressed that there were moments when they didn't bond with, or even particularly like, their children at all. It was evident that admitting these feelings made them feel ashamed.

Talking openly about these difficult issues in a women-only space offered a sense of relief, regardless of being in a mixed group of mothers and non-mothers. This demonstrates the value of employing the focus group as a method for this type of research project, as such a space can enable women to share their life experiences within a safe environment through group conversations (Dimitriadis and Kamberelis 2013; Wilkinson 1999). This was noted as particularly meaningful as such expressions of motherhood are rarely made visible culturally in stories about family, and are a taboo, socially. As argued by Shari Thurer (1994), the good mother is a cultural invention, a myth, and that most mothers feel guilt and shame about their maternal experiences in the shadow of such idealised constructions of motherhood that dominate cultural narratives. I was able to identify that the 'love spell' between mother and baby at birth is a motif adapted from prolific use in heterosexual romance narratives. The mothers in the focus groups clearly recognised these moments, and the mother–child bond, as being based in myth. As Carrie somewhat bravely stated: 'It's that whole mythology around maternal love… you can hate them [the children] more than any other person'. It's worth emphasising further how the lesbian surrogate is the only character in the texts that is depicted as having no emotional bond with the baby at the birth, which further emphasises the notion that motherhood and lesbianism are not compatible, and how a good mother must be heterosexually shaped in the narrative to be perceived by TV producers as acceptable to mainstream television audiences.

Furthermore, in relation to the baby love bond, the participants also rejected, regardless of their maternal status, race, class, or sexual orientation, the belief that authentic kinship bonds can only be formed through a genetic tie—whether that is a child produced through normative heterosexual love and natural pregnancy, or bonds with siblings and family members. Through the audience data I was able to identify how the narratives across all of the texts in focus imply that the genetic tie is symbolic of what it means to be a *real* mother (and father), a *real* child, a *real* family, which also has to be wrapped up in a white bundle, as the discussion of race, reproductive technologies and the genetic tie also revealed.

In response to these ideologies of normative family, heterosexuality, romance, whiteness and natural reproduction that were recognised in the texts, what emerged as insightful in the audience data was how meaningful attachments of love can be formed outside of the genetic bond, through a variety of kinship connections. In response to a scene in *Coronation Street* when character, Beth Tinker, delivers a line that expresses the belief that a person doesn't know real love until they've had their own child, the participants promptly discarded this notion through being able to share their own experiences of genuine and meaningful love that was not conditional on a genetic tie with a child. Many of the participants were able to talk about their love bonds outside of their romantic relationships and/or genetic children, with humans and animals which they considered part of the family. This aspect of the research

I found the most revealing, particularly as the value of the genetic tie with a child, in relation to the discourse of real family and real love, was identified as a fundamental goal throughout all of the texts selected for this project. There were some exceptions to this. Tina, the surrogate in *Coronation Street*—unlike the lesbian surrogate Brenda in *Rules of Engagement*—still fell in love with the baby, even though she was not genetically related to him. The participants believed the act of gestation and the birthing of the child created the close bond, as many of them also felt this was something they too would struggle with.

Through these discussions of more alternative forms of love, outside of genetic connections, a refusal to accept conventional notions of family was detected. What became apparent through this was the value of counter-narratives of family, which I was able to liken to the alternative kinship models that exist in urban poor, black communities and gay subcultures, which are described as fictive, or chosen families. A key research question asked: what do narratives of surrogacy represent in relation to motherhood and family? It has been made evident that the narratives of surrogacy, in the context of the value of the genetic tie, aim to perpetuate normative ideals of family through ideologies of heterosexuality, romance, whiteness and natural production—which in relation to the surrogacy storylines was positioned as the more preferable reproductive route—that shape the characterisations and narratives in the texts. However, it has transpired that the participants opposed this. Female viewers in my sample wished to see protagonists in the stories that might remain childless, and still be situated in the 'proximity to okayness, without passing some test to prove it' (Berlant 2008, 9). In this context, the test is falling pregnant naturally within a monogamous heterosexual relationship or becoming a mother through surrogacy.

Furthermore, the participants also wished to see a wider cultural acceptance and reflection of more alternative kinship structures, and to acknowledge different, but equally as valuable, forms of love that function outside of a genetic bond. The way the participants, from a variety of different subject positions, talked about how they loved their friends' children, their step siblings, or their pets—as well as their own kids—was truly reflective of how love as a concept is more complex and elastic than has been articulated. This opposes the core encoding in the texts, that the genetic tie had to be created to make a family normative and complete. It has been evidenced here that this is not the case. It is important to note that there are left-of-mainstream cultural projects that *do* reflect alternative formations of motherhood and family. However, in the popular mainstream texts with surrogacy storylines that have been examined for this project, these have not been found.

Fault Lines

What transpired as particularly illuminating through this research are two papers that explore the social constructions of infertility. Margarete Sandelowski's (1990) work which investigates women's responses to fictional representations of infertility; and Franklin's (1990) analysis of IVF narratives in popular news stories. As I have expanded on in the analysis of fertile and infertile characters across all of the texts in focus for this study, Franklin identified the winner/loser binary in how IVF news stories of childless couples are depicted in the popular media—those who get pregnant through IVF, and those who don't. The narratives, as Franklin highlights, are shaped by a discourse of desperateness. In this work Franklin also claims desperateness has two explanatory systems, the social *and* the biological, which as mentioned has been identified in this book through the participants' discussions of social failure and the stigmatisation of being infertile and/or childless by choice, which they explored through their own experiences. Where Franklin focuses on winners and losers and narrative closure through successful medical assistance, Sandelowski attends to fictional representations of infertile women in novels which she argues work to divide women. Emphasising a similar winner/loser narrative approach, Sandelowski claims through her ethnographic research of the lived experiences of women affected by infertility and her reading of fictional representations that we 'live in a cultural milieu that promotes motherhood and subverts sisterhood' (1990, 34). She was able to draw parallels between both sides of the data, primarily that voids between women are constructed as the result of reproductive (and social) dysfunction, one outcome being a lack of shared experience which causes isolation through feelings of failure, envy, rage and torment. This, Sandelowski proposes, results in conflict.

Although published almost three decades ago, both of these works have been valuable in underscoring how the articulations of infertility in the media narratives discussed in this book are purposefully constructed to create divisions between women. Despite it being argued that female characters are often shaped in opposition to each other to explore the complexities around the notion of sisterhood (Berridge and Boyle 2014).[1] I propose that this study reveals that such narrative methods *attempt* to remind women (and wider society) of their biological destiny during a time of reproductive crisis, where women are choosing alternative life paths outside of motherhood, and the configurations of family outside of the nuclear model continue to evolve. Desperate and unhappy heterosexual women struggling to overcome infertility are at the centre of these TV storylines. It is these depictions and how women are continually pitted against each other for entertainment which is most troubling. This, as has been demonstrated throughout this book, is a narrative that continues to resurface.

Drama Queens

As mentioned, the drama category was omitted from the analysis for focus. However, as has been highlighted, two significant TV programmes have since emerged which make drama an important category to consider—*The Handmaid's Tale* and *Top of the Lake: China Girl*, the latter of which takes primary focus due to its central transnational surrogacy storyline. Although *The Handmaid's Tale* does not precisely illustrate the surrogacy practice due to handmaids being forcibly impregnated and delivering babies that they are genetically related to, this text is still considered relevant due to the principal themes that shape the narrative.[2] I propose that these texts indicate a narrative shift in how the practice of surrogacy is articulated in popular culture through the drama genre. As highlighted in Chapter 1, genres boundaries blur across factual, fiction and entertainment programming, which this book has acknowledged. This hybridisation is also applicable to TV drama, especially in relation to these two programmes, as drama follows no set genre conventions as it incorporates core elements of documentary, soap opera and the sitcom. Although the development of drama as a genre cannot be expanded upon on in detail here,[3] what can be underscored is how these two programmes are dominantly influenced by soap opera techniques, primarily through the central narratives being shaped by themes of motherhood and family which also attempt to tackle issues of public concern. Such a combination produces the ideal soap opera recipe of melodrama.

Top of the Lake: China Girl and *The Handmaid's Tale* are built on melodrama's theatrical energy. The narratives of these shows encompass high emotions, startling morals, a suffering heroine and a villain—a common storyline constructed for a popular audience (Brooks 1996; Rahill 1967; L. Smith 2018). In *The Handmaid's Tale* extreme measures are taken due to a plague of infertility. The main character June and her young daughter are captured trying to flee to the safety of Canada. Her young daughter is taken away, her husband is shot. He manages to escape, but June assumes he is dead. June, and many other fertile women, are held reproductive hostage by high-ranking white couples under a fascist regime reminiscent of Nazi totalitarianism. June is repeatedly raped by 'The Commander' Fred Waterford in an attempt to impregnate her, due to the threat of *no future*. Her primary aim is to keep herself alive so she can keep her children safe.[4] In *Top of the Lake: China Girl*, a group of Thai sex workers in Sydney are illegally contracted as surrogates. Their German pimp-master 'Puss' is also the boyfriend of Mary (he is 42, she is 17), whom he is priming for prostitution. Mary's adoptive mother Julia becomes embroiled in a maternal battle with Mary's genetic mother Robin, who also happens to be the lead detective investigating the death of a pregnant Thai surrogate. Under threat is the safety of the intended parents' foetuses and Mary's moral and physical wellbeing. In addition to the classic melodramatic narrative, these shows also reveal how melodrama organises narratives through binary opposition, which John Mercer and Martin Shingler (2004) describe as Manichean, due to the genre's 'polarities of good and evil, vice and virtue, innocence and villainy' (2004, 85). Melodrama has been widely absorbed into American cinema and is viewed by drama purists as pertaining little critical value (Morse 1972). However, what these two texts demonstrate is how melodrama has widely influenced TV drama, in the form of maternal melodrama, which I propose is a more accurate description of these shows. Naomi Pfeffer describes the combination of desperation and infertility, which drive the narratives in these shows, as a 'particularly potent mix; one which forces fecund women to lease their womb, send infertile men and women scouring the world for orphans to adopt and incites some doctors into developing new techniques that subject people to many indignities' (in McNeil 1990, 204). For TV drama, the practice of surrogacy is pure maternal melodramatic gold.

However, in relation to the TV shows and Hollywood film that have been discussed throughout this book, there are some key similarities and differences in relation to the themes that have been identified which are worth emphasising. In *Top of the Lake: China Girl* there is a happy ending for Mary and her adopted mother Julia. After a period of falling off the straight line of normativity (Mary dating a pimp, Julia becoming a lesbian) both are reunited within the family home, Julia is reinserted back into a heterosexual relationship, the family unit is restored. She is no longer deemed unfit for parenthood as her desire for motherhood has heterosexualised her. This reflects the debate in Chapter 3 that argues lesbianism is just a temporary phase, the cure being penetration by a man.

What is also interesting about this resolution is that unlike the other texts explored in this project, the bond has been solidified outside of the genetic tie, which is what the participants in this project were yearning for. Hence, this heightens the importance to expand on this analysis in a more nuanced project. Another point of interest is how Mary's genetic mother Robin is removed from the family scene to enable the normative picture, much like lesbian surrogate Brenda in *Rules of Engagement*. Although Robin relinquished Mary through adoption and not surrogacy, her character performs in a similar way—she battles for the child much like Tina in *Coronation Street*.[5] This further illustrates the soap-esque maternal melodrama that shapes these texts (Brunsdon 1997; Gledhill 1987; Mumford 1991, 1995; Williams 1991). Additionally, it could be suggested, based on the findings in this book, that Robin's character has been crafted as an 'Other Mother' (Farquhar 1996) due to her deviancy as a single woman choosing a career over a relationship, who conceived a child through rape and not heterosexual love.

One distinctive difference that situates *Top of the Lake: China Girl* in opposition to the core findings in this research project, is how the articulation of transnational surrogacy impacts on the programme's final resolution. In the last episode, surrogate/sex worker ringleader 'Puss' gathers up the heavily pregnant Thai women and boards them onto a flight home, leaving the intended parents in despair. Their genetic future children disappearing off into the sunset is not the happy ending seen in the resolutions examined in this book. Puss's parting gift as the plane departs is a peculiar home video on DVD that's been left for the intended parents. The Thai surrogates are pictured playing with white babies, acting out the monetisation of the reproductive exchange by accepting wads of cash from white men. Puss's commentary throughout the footage suggests that the surrogacy arrangements were conducted to make a political statement against Western capitalism, which he claims exploits the bodies of impoverished Asian women. Puss states through his narration that: 'now the shoe is on the other foot, the tide has turned, your babies have flown away and now it's your turn to cry'.[6] This season of *Top of the Lake* was not critically well received by the media.[7] However, what this final resolution did do well is reflect the current laws in New South Wales which permit surrogates to change their minds. Through the eyes of the law they are the legal mothers. In comparison to *The Handmaid's Tale* which through austere maternal melodrama explores the more complex themes of resistance and female friendship, *Top of the Lake: China Girl* is far closer to the true spirit of melodrama through its outlandish storylines, which are more pantomime than serious drama. I propose this reflects more accurately melodrama's comic theatrical origins. I'm excited to see what a future research project exploring these two texts will reveal.

Future Work

To conclude, aside from the further analysis of the TV dramas I wish to undertake, I would like to signal new research possibilities based on this project's contributions. This will include a discussion of not just how and why as a researcher I may wish to continue the research, but how the findings that I have collated may inspire other social scientists to pick up the analytical baton, in numerous possible ways, to expand upon what has already been realised.

Firstly, inspired by Cathy J. Cohen's (1997) call for coalition politics between heterosexuality 'and everything "queer"' (1997, 438), I believe this project has highlighted how divisions between identity boundaries need to be destabilised, and that further recognition is necessary to illuminate that non-normative practices of family and reproduction exist on both sides of the hetero/homo binary. In the texts that have been analysed for this project, such family formations have not been represented. Cohen has argued that such divisions must be destabilised rather than strengthened. The narratives in these texts are doing their work to reinforce norms of family through normative notions of femininity, family, masculinity and race, which in doing so strengthens these boundaries, even if they appear, at first sight, progressive. The audience data gestures a desire for a weakening of these divides, through representation; that notions of family, motherhood and a feminine identity can transcend those which are being shaped as the ideals through the narrative conclusions. I believe that future research can be developed through exploring further the similarities that have been drawn between the representations of marginalised subjects on both sides of the heterosexual/homosexual binary, which I propose has potential to open up a new space for discussion within queer and feminist politics.

In addition, in the context of the discussion of how certain bodies are excluded from dominant representations—in relation to motherhood, reproductive technologies and family—throwing a wider analytical net outside of solely surrogacy storylines would be revealing. Therefore, further research focusing on the cultural exclusions of these bodies would be worthwhile. Such a project would explore more deeply the cultural anxieties of motherhood outside of the preferred dominant maternal poster girl of the white, middle class, heterosexual woman—specifically lesbians, the disabled and women of colour. This could further expose notions of what are considered acceptable representations of motherhood and reproduction in mainstream popular culture.

Furthermore, the representation of lesbianism and motherhood has emerged as being problematic, particularly in the context of normative notions of desirable femininity. Although this book has touched upon these issues by producing responses from lesbian and bisexual participants, it is not a lesbian-focused project. However, what *can* be highlighted is that further work is needed that addresses concerns of lesbian maternal representations more extensively. Not through textual analysis alone, but through audience reception with lesbian audiences. As one of the research questions asked, how do representations of motherhood, infertility and family reflect women's own situated experiences in the world? If motherhood and lesbianism isn't made visible, or is only shaped through certain heteronormative ideologies, then this sector of the female community is being excluded from dominant representations of family, which this research shows. Rebecca Feasey (2015) highlighted in her work with mothers examining maternal representations on TV, there has been little research exploring how these maternal audiences respond to such representations on TV and the wider media. However, in regard to the representation of lesbian motherhood, there is even less. As the female audiences in Feasey's research pointed out, there is a lack of lesbian mothers shown on popular TV shows.

Although this body of text-audience work on lesbian representation is growing[8] it is still an underdeveloped area, particularly through audience studies. As highlighted by Ruth Lewis and Julie Scanlon (2016), who have studied women's experiences of viewing lesbian representations on screen:

> Scholarly analyses of the representation of LGBTQ characters on screen are plentiful. Less plentiful are qualitative empirical studies examining audience responses to representations of LGBTQ characters on screen. Such audience studies can afford an important insight into how audiences use such representations within their lives. (2016, 3)

What has also surfaced as a prominent theme throughout the project is what I have described as the delayed conception plotline. This is an extension of the term 'delayed consummation plotline' (Scodari in Battles and Hilton-Morrow 2002, 92), where the interaction of characters in the narrative is driven by the search for a romantic relationship. In this revision, the search for love has been eclipsed by the search for a genetic child. This plotline has been a central narrative driver in all of the texts under analysis. However, as a consumer of popular culture, I have noted that such a plotline is also becoming increasingly prolific in narratives across a variety of genres, from a variety of different medias. I believe this indicates additional research outside of surrogacy storylines would contribute further to the field of maternal studies.

Finally, I feel it is imperative to emphasise that the premise of this book is not to argue for the abolishment of the family, or for the liberation of women by removing their role in biological reproduction (Firestone 1970), but to challenge the norms pervaded by the ideology of family and to make a space for alternative families, or no families at all. The 'should' in the ideology of normative kin-based families (Rapp et al. 1979) should be changed to 'shouldn't have to'. Family formations are now more diverse outside of the aspirational nuclear family model, which *should* be more widely reflected in popular culture. Furthermore, infertile subjects, as seen in the characters in the texts—or women who *choose* to live childfree—should be seen to be able to pursue alternative paths outside of normative motherhood without the anxieties and insecurities of not fitting into dominant social norms.

Notes

1. See the discussion of female friendships in *Baby Mama* (2008), *Mamma Mia* (2008) and *Bridesmaids* (2011) in Berridge and Boyle, 'I Love You, Man'.
2. A gestational surrogacy storyline materialises In Season 2. During a flash back to life prior to the enforced servitude, June's lesbian friend Moira

becomes a surrogate. This evidence of her fertility provides context for her being later apprehended to reproduce. Interestingly, as a lesbian character she is depicted as displaying a bond with the child, unlike the other lesbian characters discussed in this book.

3. For an in-depth and far more nuanced discussion of melodrama, see Gledhill and Williams, 'Melodrama Unbound'.
4. In Season 2, June has another child with her Guardian Nick, whom she falls in love with.
5. In 'Battle of the Mothers' (Season 2, Episode 6), 'Puss' turns to Robin during a confrontation and says: 'Has it ever occurred to you?' Robin: 'What?' Puss: 'That you are a surrogate too?'.
6. Although this position does reflect widespread moral debates on transnational surrogacy, this narrative resolution makes no sense. It would be highly unlikely that Thai women would undertake financial responsibility for a child that wasn't genetically theirs. Furthermore, the irony is that they too are being exploited by Puss as docile bodies—they are controlled and supervised by him.
7. This second season of *Top of the Lake* has been widely criticised across the media, described as 'out there' bizarre nonsense which is overly misogynistic. Nicholson, 'Uneven and Bizarre'. Lyons, 'Soaks in Mood'. Hogan, 'depressingly dysfunctional'.
8. See Gilbertson and Jackson, 'Hot Lesbians', Lewis and Scanlon, 'Whose sexuality?', Hallam and Marshment, 'Oranges', Mckenna, 'Queer Insistence', and Stacey, 'Stargazing'.

References

Ahmed, Sara. 2006. *Queer Phenomenology: Orientations, Objects, Others*. London: Routledge.

Ahmed, Sara. 2010. *The Promise of Happiness*. Durham: Duke University Press.

Baby Mama. 2008. Directed and Written by Michael McCullers. Film. Universal City, CA: Universal Pictures.

Battles, Kathleen, and Wendy Hilton-Morrow 2002. "Gay Characters in Conventional Spaces: Will and Grace and the Situation Comedy Genre." *Critical Studies in Media Communication* 19 (1): 87–105.

Berlant, Lauren. 2008. *The Female Complaint*. Durham: Duke University Press.

Berridge, Susan, and Karen Boyle. 2014. "I Love You, Man: Gendered Narratives of Friendship in Contemporary Hollywood Movies." *Feminist Media Studies* 14 (3): 353–368.

Bridesmaids. 2011. Directed by Paul Feig. Written by Kristen Wiig and Annie Mumolo. Film. Universal City, California: Universal Pictures.

Brooks, Peter. 1996. *The Melodramatic Imagination*. New Haven: Yale University Press.

Brundson, Charlotte. 1997. *Screen Tastes: Soap Opera to Satellite Dishes*. London: Routledge.

Bruzzi, Stella. 2001. "Docusoaps." In *The Television Genre Book*, edited by Glenn Creeber, Toby Miller, and John Tulloch. London: BFI.

Carroll, Noel. 1996. *Theorizing the Moving Image*. Cambridge: Cambridge University Press.

Cohen, Cathy J. 1997. "Punks, Bulldaggers, and Welfare Queens: The Radical Potential of Queer Politics?" *GLQ: A Journal of Lesbian and Gay Studies* 3 (4): 437–465.

Coronation Street. 1960–present. Created by Tony Warren. TV Programme. Manchester: ITV.

Dimitriadis, Greg, and George Kamberelis. 2013. *Focus Groups*. New York: Routledge.

Farquhar, Dion. 1996. *The Other Machine: Discourse and Reproductive Technologies*. London: Routledge.

Feasey, Rebecca. 2015. *Mothers on Mothers: Maternal Readings of Popular Television*. Edinburgh: Edinburgh University Press.

Firestone, Shulamith. 1970. *Dialectic of Sex: The Case for a Feminist Revolution*. New York: Naomi Wolf.

Foucault, Michel. 1977. *Discipline and Punish: The Birth of the Prison*. London: Penguin.

Franklin, Sarah. 1990. "Deconstructing Desperateness': The Social Construction of Infertility in Popular Representations of New Reproductive Technologies." In *The New Reproductive Technologies*, edited by Maureen McNeil. London: Palgrave Macmillan.

Giuliana & Bill. 2009–2014. Executively Produced by Alastair Surprise, Robert Sizemore. TV Programme. Los Angeles, CA: E!

Gledhill, Christine. 1987. "Speculations on the Relationship Between Soap Opera and Melodrama." *Quarterly Review of Film and Video* 14 (1–2): 103–124.

Gorton, Kristyn. 2009. *Media Audiences*. Edinburgh: Edinburgh University Press.

Grey's Anatomy. 2005–present. "Fear (Of the Unknown)" Season 10, Episode 24. Directed by Bill D'Elia. Written by Shonda Rhimes. May 15, 2014. TV Programme. New York: ABC.

Halberstam, Judith. 2011. *The Queer Art of Failure*. Durham: Duke University Press.

Kuhn, Annette. 1992. *Women's Pictures: Feminism and Cinema*. 2nd ed. London: Verso.

Lam, Carla. 2015. *New Reproductive Technologies and Disembodiment*. 1st ed. Abingdon: Routledge.

Lewis, Ruth, and Judith Scanlon. 2016. "Whose sexuality is it anyway? Women's experiences of viewing lesbians on screen." *Feminist Media Studies* 17 (6): 1005–1021.

Mamma Mia! 2008. Directed by Phyllida Lloyd. Written by Kristen Catherine Johnson. Film. Universal City, California: Universal Pictures.

McNeil, Maureen. 1990. *The New Reproductive Technologies*. London: Palgrave Macmillan.

Mercer, John, and Martin Shingler. 2004. *Melodrama: Genre, Style and Sensibility*. New York: Wallflower Press.
Morse, David. 1972. "Aspects of Melodrama." *Monogram* 4: 16–17.
Mumford, Laura. 1991. "Plotting Paternity: Looking for Dad on Daytime Soaps." *Genders* 12: 45–61.
Mumford, Laura. 1995. *Love and Ideology in the Afternoon: Soap Opera, Women, and Television Genre*. Bloomington: Indiana University Press.
Oliver, Kelly. 2012. *Knock Me Up, Knock Me Down*. New York: Columbia University Press.
Packer, Vin. 1952. *Spring Fire*. New York: Gold Medal.
Rahill, Frank. 1967. *World of Melodrama*. University Park, PA: Pennsylvania State University Press.
Rapp, Rayna, Ross Ellen, and Renate Bridenthal. 1979. "Examining Family History." *Feminist Studies* 5 (1): 174.
Roberts, Dorothy. 1995. "The Genetic Tie." *The University of Chicago Law Review* 62 (1): 209–273.
Roberts, Dorothy. 1996. "Race and the New Reproduction." *Faculty Scholarship at Penn Law*. 1154.
Roberts, Dorothy. 2000. *Killing the Black Body: Race, Reproduction, and the Meaning of Liberty*. New York: Vintage Books.
Rules of Engagement. 2007–2013. Created by Tom Hertz. TV Programme. New York: CBS.
Sandelowski, Margarete. 1990. "Fault Lines: Infertility and Imperiled Sisterhood." *Feminist Studies* 16 (1): 33.
Smith, James L. 2018. *Melodrama*. 2nd ed. Oxon: Routledge.
Smith, Murray. 1995. *Engaging Characters: Fiction, Emotion and the Cinema*. Oxford: Clarendon Press.
The Handmaid's Tale. 2017–present. Created by Bruce Miller. Written by Margaret Atwood. TV Programme. Channel 4.
The New Normal. 2012–2013. Created by Elodie Keene, Max Winkler, Ryan Murphy. TV Programme. New York: NBC.
Throsby, Karen. 2004. *When IVF Fails: Feminism, Infertility and the Negotiation of Normal*. Basingstoke: Palgrave.
Thurer, Shari. 1994. *Myths of Motherhood: How Culture Reinvents the Good Mother*. Boston: Houghton Mifflin Harcourt.
Top of the Lake: China Girl. 2017. Directed by Jane Campion. Written by Jane Campion, Gerard Lee. TV Programme. London: BBC2.
Warner, Michael. 1999. *The Trouble with Normal*. Cambridge, MA: Harvard University Press.
Williams, Linda. 1991. "Film Bodies: Gender, Genre, and Excess." *Film Quarterly* 44 (4): 2–13.
Wilkinson, Sue. 1999. "Focus Groups: A Feminist Method." *Psychology of Women Quarterly* 23 (2): 221–244.

Appendices

Appendix A: Glossary of Terms

BME—Black, Minority, and Ethnic.

Commercial surrogate—a surrogate is compensated beyond medical expenses for a couple or person. Usually, in this arrangement, the surrogate doesn't use her own eggs.

Embryo transfer—embryos are placed in the uterus with the hope of creating a pregnancy.

Gestational surrogate—similar to a commercial surrogate, the gestational surrogate is usually compensated beyond medical expenses for a couple or person, but not always, as it is dependent on the country and the state. However, gestational surrogacy means the surrogate doesn't use her own eggs, but either the intended parent's embryo, created through their genetic matter or with the help of a donor/s.

Intended mother (IM)—the woman who enters into an agreement to be the legal mother to a child born through surrogacy.

Intended parents (IPs)—a man and a woman, or a same-sex couple, who enter into an agreement with a surrogate with a contract who under the terms agreed will be the parents to the child. Usually one

L. Le Vay, *Surrogacy and the Reproduction of Normative Family on TV*, Palgrave Studies in Science and Popular Culture,
https://doi.org/10.1007/978-3-030-17570-2

of the intended parents has a genetic connection to the child, but not always.

IVF cycle—eggs are retrieved at point of maturation and fertilised in the IVF lab to create embryos.

LGTBQ—Lesbian, Gay, Transsexual, Bisexual, Queer.

Parental order—is a legal document that transfers the legal rights from the birth mother in Britain to the intended parents, when a surrogate is used.

Traditional surrogate—this type of surrogacy involves the woman using her own eggs, which she fertilises through either IVF or artificial insemination.

Transnational surrogacy—is a form of medical tourism when intended parents turn to the Global South to engage a foreign surrogate labourer.

Appendix B: Description of the Texts

Genre: Drama

The Handmaid's Tale *(2017–Present)*

The Handmaid's Tale is a contemporary re-working of Margaret Atwood's (1985) dystopian novel, which tells the story of a fundamentalist regime in America who apprehend fertile women due to plummeting birth rates as a result of widespread infertility. This new administration makes them the property of the state to reproduce.

The narrative follows the main character June as she tries to escape to find her young daughter who was also captured. In the second season, the narrative extends beyond the original book. June falls in love with her Guardian and falls pregnant with his child. At the end of the season the newborn is transported through the underground communities to safety. Safe in this knowledge, June turns back to find her daughter.

Top of the Lake: China Girl *(2017)*

The primary storyline in *Top of the Lake: China Girl* revolves around detective Robin Griffin who is investigating the death of a pregnant Thai sex worker in Sydney. During the enquiry, Robin makes contact with her

17-year-old biological daughter Mary who she's not seen since birth. Mary is romantically involved with an older man who is the mastermind of a transnational surrogacy foetus heist to make a political statement. Mary's adoptive mother Julia becomes embroiled in a maternal battle with Mary's genetic mother Robin.

Genre: Reality TV

Giuliana & Bill *(E! 2009–2014)*
Giuliana & Bill is a popular American reality TV show that follows the lives of E! News anchor, Giuliana, and her husband Bill Rancic. The show is driven by the couple's desire to have a child. Giuliana suffers several miscarriages and failed IVF treatment. She also discovers she has breast cancer, which she survives. The couple contract gestational surrogate, Delphine, to carry their genetic child. Their son Duke is born during Season 5 (2012).

Genre: Sitcom

The New Normal *(NBC, 2012–2013)*
The New Normal is an American sitcom that tells the story of LA-based homosexual couple Bryan and David as they contract single mother Goldie, a waitress from Ohio, to be their surrogate. Goldie and her young 8-year-old daughter Shania move into their home during the pregnancy. The cast includes Goldie's grandmother Jane, and Bryan's assistant and best friend, Rocky. The show was cancelled after one season.

Rules of Engagement *(CBS, 2007–2013)*
This American sitcom follows the lives of two heterosexual couples and their single heterosexual friend. The focus of this show for this project is the surrogacy storyline, in relation to married couple Jeff and Audrey. The couple are unable to conceive a child, naturally, due to Audrey's infertility, therefore they engage Jeff's best friend, Brenda, who is a lesbian, to be the surrogate. Due to pregnancy sickness, Brenda moves into the couple's home for the duration of her pregnancy. At the end of the season, during the last ever show, Brenda gives birth. Soon after, Audrey finds out she is pregnant, naturally.

Genre: Soap

Coronation Street *(ITV, 1960–Present)*
A surrogacy storyline emerged in 2012, which ran until June 2013. Couple Gary and Izzy were unable to have a child of their own due to Izzy's disability disallowing her to carry a foetus to term. Their neighbour, Tina, needed money to pay of a large debt. Izzy's father Owen pays off Tina's debt under agreed surrogacy expenses, which is legally permitted in Britain. In addition, Owen also provides Tina and her partner Tommy with somewhere to live during her pregnancy. However, after giving birth to a boy, Jake, Tina bonds with the child and refuses to relinquish him to his genetic parents. In Britain, as the woman who gives birth to the child, Tina is the legal birth mother, despite not having a genetic tie. After weeks of feuding, Tina eventually decides to give Jake to Izzy and Gary.

Genre: Film

Baby Mama *(Universal, 2008)*
Successful businesswoman Kate has been unable to find Mr. Right, and has been told by doctors she is infertile due to having an abnormal uterus. Kate is desperate for a child, so she contracts Angie from a surrogacy agency. Angie and her common-law husband, Carl, lie about the pregnancy as a scam to get paid the $10,000 fee. Angie breaks up with Carl and moves in with Kate. Angie then discovers, to her surprise, that she *is* actually pregnant, but with her and Carl's baby. Kate falls in love with Rob, who she meets through work. Despite falling out over the fake pregnancy, Kate is with Angie when she goes into labour, where she too discovers she is pregnant. The women remain friends.

Appendix C: Description of Focus Groups

Description of the Focus Group Structure

The session was divided into three sections: texts-in-action (Wood 2009), a group discussion of the texts, followed by game Agree/Disagree (Kitzinger 1994). The texts-in-action section of the group was when the participants were observed by the researcher viewing a number of clips from texts selected for analysis, as outlined in

Appendix B. The participants were given paper and pens if they wished to make notes and scribbles. The group interview was led by semi-structured questions, to help the participants discuss the clips in the order that they were viewed. This was then followed by a game called Agree/Disagree, which is where the groups were encouraged to put statements pulled from the clips into two columns. This method had been tested in a previous project.

List of Participants

Group 1—Mixed mothers

Name	*Age*	*Ethnicity*	*Occupation*	*Social class*	*Sexuality*
Jackie	39	White American	Jewellery designer	Middle-class	Bisexual
Carla	42	White British	Acupuncturist	Middle-class	Heterosexual
Sonja	42	Anglo-Indian	Picture editor	Middle-class	Heterosexual
Carrie	43	Black Canadian	Secondary school teacher	Middle-class	Heterosexual
Nadra	38	White Irish	PR consultant	Working-class	Heterosexual
Sally	41	White British	Art restorer	Middle-class	Heterosexual

Group 2—Non-mothers

Name	*Age*	*Ethnicity*	*Occupation*	*Social class*	*Sexuality*
Laura	37	White British	DJ	Working-class	Heterosexual
Tara	38	White British	HE outreach officer	Middle-class	Heterosexual
Rebecca	37	Anglo Indian	TV news producer	Middle-class	Heterosexual
Paula	22	Black British	Musician	Working-class	Heterosexual
Charlie	27	White British	International relocation manager	Middle-class	Heterosexual
Rachel	41	Black British	Poet	Working-class	Lesbian
Tanya	37	Anglo Indian	Events manager	Middle-class	Heterosexual

Group 3—Pre-mothers

Name	*Age*	*Ethnicity*	*Social class*
Rhian	18	Anglo Indian	Working-class
Fay	17	White British	Working-class
Rose	18	Turkish Cypriot	Working-class
Claire	18	White British	Working-class
Candice	17	White British	Working-class
Jess	18	Black British	Working-class

Index

L. Le Vay, *Surrogacy and the Reproduction of Normative Family on TV*, Palgrave Studies in Science and Popular Culture, https://doi.org/10.1007/978-3-030-17570-2

Kolibri 360 GmbH
Ferdinand-Jühlke-Straße 7
99095 Erfurt, Deutschland
produktsicherheit@kolibri360.de